BIRTH AFTER CAESAREAN

Jenny Lesley

COMMUNITY FUND
Lottery money making a difference

Supported by the Community Fund
Published by AIMS
© AIMS March 2004
ISBN 978 1 874413 17 2

Acknowledgements

Jenny Lesley would like to thank Gina Lowdon and Debbie Chippington Derrick for their incredibly generous support, hard work and encouragement without which this booklet could never have been written.

AIMS would like to thank Jenny for undertaking this project, and Gina and Debbie for all their work. We are also extremely grateful to Rosemary Mander who did the initial research review. Our discussions with Rosemary were very valuable and helped us to develop the framework for this book.

About this booklet

This booklet aims to provide information about choices, suggest ways in which a vaginal birth after a caesarean can be made more likely and inform women about their rights and where to find support.

Throughout, vaginal birth after caesarean is referred to as VBAC (pronounced *vee-back*). Other terms commonly used include VBA2Cs (vaginal birth after two caesareans) and HBAC (home birth after caesarean). For an explanation of any other terms used please refer to the Glossary on page 67.

Contents

What's So Good About VBAC?	1
Why Don't You Just Have Another Caesarean?	3
Just how safe are caesareans?	5
Are risks increased for multiple caesareans?	7
Are there risks of caesarean for the baby?	9
What about "once a caesarean, always a caesarean"?	9
What About Caesarean Scar Rupture?	11
Is there anything that makes scar rupture more likely?	12
What are the signs of rupture and what can be done about it?	14
What Are My Chances of Having a VBAC?	14
Research and me	15
Comparing VBAC With Elective Repeat Caesarean	16
You May Have Heard That You Can't Have a VBAC When...	18
Your previous caesarean was for 'failure to progress'/fetal distress/a small pelvis	18
Your baby is too big	19
You have had more than one previous caesarean	20
Your baby is in the breech position	21
You are carrying twins or triplets	22
It is too soon after your caesarean	22
Your scar is not a lower segment horizontal scar	23
You're too old, too fat, etc	23
Making VBAC More Likely	24
Thinking about previous birth experiences	24
Finding support for VBAC	25
Finding good midwifery support	28
Considering other birth supporters	30
Considering a home birth	31

Considering a birth centre or midwife-led unit	33
Considering induction	33
Deciding when to go into hospital and how long to labour	36
Considering how the baby should best be monitored	37
Using birth pools or 'home from home' rooms	39
Considering the need for a cannula	40
Encouraging the baby into a good position for labour ('optimal fetal positioning')	40
Using upright positions for labour	41
Thinking about pain relief	42

Planning Your VBAC — 42

VBAC Birth Reports	44
Theo's birth - a vaginal birth after a previous classical incision caesarean – *Sarah Carrek*	44
Jenna's birth story, a VBA2Cs – *Rach Pritchard*	46
Against medical advice, an underwater home VBAC – *Caroline L Spear*	50
Triumph of hope over experience – a HWBA3Cs – *Jenny Lesley*	54

If You Do Need Another Caesarean — 60

Are there advantages to a repeat caesarean?	61
Making the most of a caesarean birth	62
Caesarean Birth Report: Danny's birth story – *Joanna Ashburner*	64

Glossary — 67

References — 70

VBAC Research — 74

Further Reading — 78

Online Resources and Information — 83

Further Support and Information — 85

What's So Good About VBAC?

Some women come away from their caesarean adamant that, next time, they will give birth vaginally. They feel they have been deprived of their birthright and another caesarean would only be acceptable should the health of their baby be under serious threat.

Other women might be feeling very unsure about how to have their next baby. They might have enjoyed their caesarean birth experience. Or might have felt there was little choice. Or might have had a really difficult birth and not want to repeat that experience again or risk it ending in sudden surgery.

It can be hard to hear that there are advantages for mother and baby in having a vaginal birth. Sometimes this can feel like a criticism of you and your previous birth choices. Thinking about some of these issues might stir up feelings of guilt or sadness or anger. If you need support as you think through these decisions then it might help to go to the end of this book and make contact with some of the groups and individuals listed. There is no value judgement intended in this book against those who choose caesarean birth or whose birth experience ends with caesarean.

As a woman or partner, looking at your options for future births you have a right to accurate, unbiased information. To present VBAC and caesarean births as an equal choice with no differences in health outcomes for mothers and babies would not be accurate or unbiased. Of course there will be situations and factors, both medical and personal, which will tip the balance of risk in one direction or another for you as an individual and which only you can judge. Birth choices are very personal and very individual. All this booklet aims to do is to ensure that you have accurate information and access to support so you can make choices with which you are comfortable.

When women were asked on an email support group how their VBAC experience was different from their previous caesarean birth some of the responses were:

- ♦ I felt in control of my labour, birth and body.
- ♦ There was a sense of peace with myself.

- I had an overwhelming feeling of "I told you I could do it!"
- It felt like a natural process rather than an appointment.
- I had a feeling of completion, a sense of achievement.
- I felt like a proper woman with VBAC.
- It was great to go home so soon.
- I was able to feed comfortably.
- I could cuddle up to my husband and toddler and share the baby.
- I had a birth he was part of instead of standing, shocked, on the sidelines.
- I went out to order a sofa the next day.
- I wasn't crying every time I coughed or sneezed.
- I was able to drive to the supermarket as soon as I wanted to.
- I didn't have to feel like a "patient" people felt sorry for.
- I could pick up my baby myself whenever he needed me.
- The older children weren't relegated to visitor status; I was within hours.
- Sex without pain was possible so much sooner.
- I had had a baby...and I could walk!

Of course not all women who are intending to have a VBAC will have one. Some will have another caesarean and some will be happy with that labour and that result, and others won't. Not all women who have a VBAC are necessarily happy with their vaginal birth experience. No-one can promise you a particular experience or say how you will feel about it, any more than they could first time around.

Overall most women who decide to VBAC do have a VBAC, although as you will see later different 'success' rates are often quoted. It also seems true to say that most who do have a VBAC are pleased with that experience. For many it will restore confidence and faith in themselves, and help them towards a sense of peace and acceptance of the previous caesarean birth.

Babies benefit from being born vaginally. They are usually born at full term, when they are ready. This makes them less likely to need special care for respiratory distress (breathing problems) or because they were 'small for dates'.

Babies who have experienced labour benefit from the surge of hormones called catecholamines which are released in the baby's body during labour and which prepare the baby for birth. These hormones help to clear the baby's lungs so that he/she can breathe, they speed up the metabolism and ensure a rich supply of blood to the heart and brain. It is these hormones which keep the baby awake for some time after birth so that the baby can bond with his mother and have his first breastfeed.

The baby who is born vaginally is much more likely to be breastfed as it makes early and frequent feeding easier – although of course many caesarean babies are breastfed too. Vaginally born babies tend to receive more attention in the early weeks of life as their mothers do not have to recover from surgery.

Women who give birth vaginally usually recover more quickly, are less likely to suffer infections and more likely to bond with their babies more quickly. There are other benefits too which you will discover as we look at the risks of caesarean birth.

> "I needed to prove to myself that my body was really capable of giving birth. I needed to feel whole again – I had lost faith in my body after having the c-section. Although logically I knew the caesarean hadn't been my fault, emotionally I had still blamed my body for not performing up to the required standards. I knew my body could do it if given a chance and I didn't want any surgery that would have been unnecessary."
>
> – Helen, HBAC

Why Don't You Just Have Another Caesarean?

If you and your caesarean-born baby are both healthy you might face some surprise or even hostility when telling friends, family or some health professionals that you are considering a VBAC. You might even be feeling unsure or angry about the idea yourself, particularly if you have had a previous difficult birth experience.

AIMS — Association for Improvements in the Maternity Services

Given the large, and growing, numbers of women who have caesarean section births in the United Kingdom many people assume that this is as safe or even safer than vaginal birth. There are also some popular myths that caesarean birth is pain-free, protects the woman from future incontinence and that there is a rule: "once a caesarean always a caesarean".

Some parents might have found the caesarean a calm and a happy start to parenthood. They may have felt fully consulted and involved in all the decisions, that the caesarean was necessary and easy to accept under the circumstances, and that being involved at close hand in a surgical operation was interesting and exciting.

> "It was so peaceful. Our music was playing, they told us what they were doing and when. The baby wasn't removed from theatre, they weighed her in front of us and I breastfed within the hour in the recovery room. We really felt involved in the birth."
>
> **– Elaine, after 3rd Caesarean**

Whilst it is true that some women are very satisfied with their caesarean birth experience, it is also common for women to feel cheated or even traumatised afterwards. You may feel that your caesarean was unnecessary and wonder whether it could have been prevented. On the other hand, you might believe that your caesarean was the best option for you and your baby, but still wonder what it would have been like to have given birth without surgery.

However routine it might be in some hospitals to offer elective section for future babies, for many women a repeat caesarean is not "just another caesarean".

> "Because my two elder children were born, their birthdays are two of the most wonderful days of my life, but I am sad to say I did not give birth to them. They were unnecessarily extracted from my abdomen. I had no input into their births. I was immobile, drugged, cut. I didn't feel them coming out of my body. My husband played no active part in their births. We were onlookers in a medical circus. I will always mourn their deliveries a little, even as I celebrate their births."
>
> **– Rach, VBA2C**

Similarly, fathers or partners may have a variety of feelings about the previous caesarean birth – some might feel they were helpless bystanders, as the birth became a roller coaster of distressing events. They might feel that staff took over and decisions were taken on which they were not consulted. Some might feel sad or angry and feel that they 'failed' to protect their partner.

Many women who have had a previous caesarean would not agree with the popular view that caesarean birth is the pain-free option. Many research studies which compare "morbidity" (feeling unwell, having unwanted side-effects and/or complications) of caesarean with women's well-being after vaginal birth, fail to collect information on post-operative pain.

Medical research also rarely considers longer-term outcomes, including long-term pain and feelings of disfigurement, let alone what may be considered the lesser difficulties of day-to-day life. The longer recovery time and the practical restrictions, like being unable to drive, carry your baby about for long periods, or not being able to cuddle your older child easily, are usually disregarded.

Concerns about the safety of VBAC are common. Women can find themselves at odds with the medical establishment, with the woman sure in her heart that VBAC is the right option for her and her baby, but facing a doctor or midwife who seems to be very anxious or uncertain about her and the baby's safety. When this happens it is easy to become demoralised and to forget that a VBAC can be considered the norm – a physiological birth with all its possibilities.

Perhaps the issue of safety should be turned on its head and we should ask ourselves about the safety of caesareans.

Just how 'safe' are caesareans?

It is often difficult to find complete, reliable and unbiased information on the risks of caesarean section. This is partly because the information that is available tends to relate to short-term problems that may occur during the operation or during the early postnatal days in hospital. As explained above, longer-term problems tend to be ignored, as they are difficult and costly to follow-up and record.

Some doctors may be more at ease with the risks of caesarean than the uncertainties of vaginal birth. It is from doctors that most women get their initial information about birth after caesarean. However, when compared with an uncomplicated vaginal birth, a 'routine' caesarean carries greater risks of complications.

Risks of caesarean section include: infection, haemorrhage (internal bleeding), embolism (blood clots in the circulation), damage to the bowel or bladder during the operation, depression (PND), posttraumatic stress disorder (PTSD), and complications from the anaesthetic (see AIMS' occasional paper, *Risks of Caesarean Sections*, page 81).

There is an increase in cases of endometritis (an infection of the lining of the uterus) in women who have had a caesarean and this may be a contributory cause of the finding that women who have had caesareans are more likely to have difficulty in conceiving more children.[1]

Having a repeat caesarean also increases the likelihood of your needing an emergency hysterectomy (removal of the uterus). A review of VBAC literature from the 1980s found that the rate of hysterectomy due to caesarean scar rupture was 0.06%, whereas the rate reported for 'obstetric haemorrhage' after caesarean section was more than ten times greater at 0.7%.[2]

Women and their families sometimes worry about their risk of dying during childbirth. Maternal death is now very rare in affluent countries – the numbers are so small they are usually measured by numbers of deaths per 100,000 women having babies. Most of these happen when there is already a known problem that makes the pregnancy complicated or an unusual problem develops during birth. Although your risk of dying during a caesarean is tiny, it is still greater than if you are having a vaginal birth:

> "The rate of maternal death associated with caesarean section (approximately 4 per 10,000 births) is four times that associated with all types of vaginal birth (1 per 10,000 births). The maternal death rate associated with elective repeat caesarean section (around 2 per 10,000 births), although lower than that associated with caesarean sections overall, is still twice the rate associated with all vaginal

deliveries, and nearly four times the mortality rate associated with normal vaginal birth (0.5 per 10,000 births)."

– Enkin et al[3]

Women can be very frightened when a doctor tells them that if they opt for VBAC their uterus might rupture and they could die, which is highly unlikely since:

"... no study in the VBAC literature has recorded a maternal death attributable to VBAC..."

– **Henci Goer, Childbirth Educator and Doula**[4]

Are risks increased for multiple caesareans?

There are substantial numbers of women in the UK who have had four or more caesareans, and at least one who has recently had her seventh, without suffering any ill-effects but, especially if you are considering having a large family, you might want to know that there are certain risks which increase with each caesarean.

Different people produce varying amounts of scar tissue as a response to surgery. Whereas some seem to produce very little, others are left with adhesions, which can cause problems for future operations. It is also not uncommon for adhesions to cause women to feel sensations of stretching, pulling and/or release during pregnancy following a caesarean as their uterus expands. Scar tissue can also make future caesarean (and other) operations more difficult to perform, occasionally leading to damage to the bladder.

The other main area of additional risk to women having multiple caesareans involves the placenta. Placenta praevia is a condition where the placenta lies across or very close to the cervix, the opening of the uterus. A placenta praevia will usually be seen at an ultrasound scan and will mean a vaginal birth cannot take place safely and a caesarean will be necessary. A low-lying placenta found at an early ultrasound scan need not necessarily be a cause for alarm as in most cases the placenta will move away from the cervix as the uterus expands. Placenta praevia can only be diagnosed with confidence during a scan in late pregnancy.

Once you have had one caesarean your risk of placenta praevia in a subsequent pregnancy more than doubles.[4] Although placenta praevia is a rare condition, which only occurs in just over 0.5% of all pregnancies,[3] it can be extremely serious. It can cause bleeding in pregnancy and, in some cases, miscarriage and stillbirth.

The risk of having a placenta accreta also increases. Placenta accreta is where the placenta grows into the lining of the uterus or into the caesarean scar tissue. This condition cannot be detected by ultrasound and is usually only a problem following the birth of the baby when the placenta does not come away as it should. This generally results in a manual removal of the placenta in an operating theatre, where complications can be dealt with if necessary. In extremely rare cases the placenta may be so embedded that attempts to remove it can result in serious haemorrhage, which can be life-threatening.

For the unlucky few with a placenta praevia, the risk of the praevia also being placenta accreta increases with the number of caesareans a woman has had. A placenta praevia accreta can be life threatening to mother and baby and can result in hysterectomy in order to prevent the mother bleeding to death.

Although the risk of having a placenta praevia remains small, one study has shown that when it does occur, the risk of the placenta praevia also being a placenta accreta increases from 5% in an unscarred uterus to 24% with one scar, to 40% with two scars and 67% with four scars. The same study showed that when women had both these conditions 82% of the women who had had a previous caesarean required a hysterectomy.[5]

Although the risks are very small; you are more likely to suffer from these placental problems after a caesarean and the risk of having both placenta praevia and accreta increases with each caesarean, as does the risk of needing a hysterectomy, which is far greater than a woman with an unscarred uterus.

Not all health professionals seem to explain the way these risks increase with each subsequent caesarean especially when promoting the safety of a repeat caesarean, but they may be worth considering carefully if you plan to have several children.

"A caesarean section casts a shadow over the rest of a woman's reproductive life...caesareans are neither safe nor easy"
– Henci Goer, Childbirth Educator and Doula[4]

Are there risks of caesarean for the baby?

In most cases a first caesarean is carried out when the baby is believed to be at risk, and indeed lives have undoubtedly been saved and health problems avoided by this operation. However, caesarean birth is not risk-free for the baby. Babies born by caesarean section, particularly if they have not had the benefit of experiencing labour contractions, are at greater risk of suffering breathing difficulties, both at birth[6] and later in life.[7]

Research has shown that the risk of a baby needing help with breathing when born by caesarean reduces with each week of continued pregnancy. This study also found that some babies were delivered by elective caesarean at 37-38 weeks simply because the mother had had a previous caesarean, instead of 39 weeks onwards, when their risk would have been so much lower.[8]

Babies are also occasionally cut by the surgeon's scalpel at the time of their caesarean birth. Although the incidence of this is not known as many cases are not reported, one study has put it at almost 2%.[9] Babies can suffer bruising too, just as they can in a difficult vaginal delivery, and it has been known for babies to suffer broken bones during their caesarean birth.

For those who would like more detailed information on the risks of caesarean birth. The AIMS occasional paper *Risks of Caesarean Sections* (see page 81) also covers risks to the baby.

What about "once a caesarean, always a caesarean"?

As for the notion "once a caesarean, always a caesarean" – this has never been normal practice in the UK. When EB Craigin wrote this in 1916,[10] he was arguing against doing a first caesarean. At that time maternal death rates from caesarean section were still very high, and he was concerned about overuse of new technology.

The caesarean section rate was under 2% and the operation was usually only carried out on women for whom vaginal birth was not possible, for example in severe cases of rickets. Also the type of cut that was made in the uterus was a high vertical one, a classical incision. There were no antibiotics at that time and many women suffered post-operative infections, consequently the rate of uterine rupture in any following pregnancy was high and often catastrophic.

As surgical techniques improved and antibiotics became more widely available, caesarean section became much safer, and the 'lower segment transverse incision' that is used today posed a much smaller risk for future pregnancies. This uses a horizontal cut much lower down in the uterus.

> "As study after study has shown, it rarely gives way, and when it does, the separation is usually like opening a zipper: neat, bloodless and benign."
>
> — **Henci Goer, Childbirth Educator and Doula**[4]

The widely respected publication *Effective Care in Pregnancy and Childbirth*, brings together good quality research evidence on healthcare interventions in maternity care from all over the world. It is written mostly by researchers and healthcare professionals, and is written mainly for medical practitioners and caregivers in maternity care, although some consumers may find it helpful too.

Although the background information in this book is extremely informative, the evidence has been updated since the book was written and is now available within The Cochrane Library.

The updated maternity care reviews produced by the Pregnancy and Childbirth Group are available electronically, updated every two years, and are now accessible via the internet (see page 84). A much smaller publication *A Guide to Effective Care in Pregnancy and Childbirth*, summarises the findings in an easily accessible form. Last published in 2000, it states:

> "Overall, attempted vaginal birth for women with a single previous low transverse caesarean section is associated with a lower risk of complications for both mother and baby than routine repeat caesarean section."
>
> — Enkin et al[3]

What About Caesarean Scar Rupture?

No woman who is thinking about having a VBAC can do so for long without coming up against the question of whether the scar on her uterus will be strong enough to support pregnancy and labour. It is this aspect of VBAC which seems to cause the most anxiety for many doctors and midwives and these concerns are often passed on to women.

The safety of VBAC and the risks of caesarean scar rupture are much debated and the subject of numerous research studies. However the widely respected book, *A Guide to Effective Care in Pregnancy and Childbirth*, concludes:

> "A planned vaginal birth after a previous caesarean section should be recommended for women whose first caesarean section was by lower segment transverse incision, and who have no other indication for caesarean section in the present pregnancy."
>
> – Enkin et al[3]

Indeed there is now a lot of evidence supporting the safety of VBAC. Despite this, *The National Sentinel Caesarean Section Audit Report* found that of women who had a repeat caesarean, only 44% were reported to have been offered a 'trial of labour', and at least one hospital was failing to offer VBAC to 92% of women with a history of caesarean section.[11]

Despite the very low risks of rupture, many doctors and some midwives still talk about VBAC as a 'trial of labour' or even 'trial of scar'. This language is very frightening for some women. It presupposes rupture; it undermines our intention to birth our babies ourselves without problems.

Part of the problem is that many research studies don't differentiate between true uterine rupture (which can be a serious, life-threatening event), and caesarean scar dehiscence. Scar dehiscence is where some or all of the layers of the uterine wall separate without causing many problems for mother, baby and/or the progress of labour and vaginal birth.

The most commonly quoted rate of caesarean scar rupture in the UK is around

0.5% or 1 in 200. Unfortunately many women understand this to mean that they have around a 1 in 200 chance of losing their baby, their uterus or their life. This is simply not the case.

> "Fortunately, the true rupture is rare in modern obstetrics, despite the increase in caesarean section rates, and serious sequelae [consequences] are even more rare. Although often considered to be the most common cause of uterine rupture, previous caesarean section is a factor in less than half the reported cases."
>
> – Enkin et al[3]

Depending on which study you look at you will find rates of true, complete rupture ranging from 0.09 to 0.8% for singleton babies born to mothers with one previous lower segment scar.[3]

Is there anything that makes scar rupture more likely?

There is concern about using drugs to induce or accelerate labour, particularly the prostaglandin gel pessaries or tablets used for many inductions. There is good evidence that this could increase the chances of rupture[12] but we simply can't tell how many of the small number of ruptures that do occur do so in women who have been induced as opposed to women in spontaneous labour.

Prostaglandins only came into widespread use in the 1980s so many of the research studies predate them (see Considering Induction page 33 for more information).

There has been concern voiced recently about whether there is an increase in rupture caused by the way in which the uterus is sewn up during caesarean section. Most surgeons in the UK use a double-layer closure but a single-layer closure is more common in the USA, where some health professionals are no longer accepting women for VBAC unless they have documented proof of a double-layer closure. Although there is concern, the evidence is weak and contradictory.

The majority of surgeons in this country use the double-layer technique and until there is further evidence about the safety of the single-layer technique, this is likely to remain the case.[13]

What are the signs of rupture and what can be done about it?

Serious cases of caesarean scar rupture are so rare that there is little information on what women and their health carers should be watching out for.

Symptoms of uterine separation may include all, some, or none of the following: abdominal pain, vaginal bleeding, a rise in pulse followed by a drop in blood pressure, baby in distress, swelling over the area of the scar, shock, fever.

Severe abdominal pain, particularly between contractions, and which may be felt despite an epidural, has warned of scar rupture in some cases. However, abdominal pain or tenderness around the area of the scar are unreliable signs of a possible rupture since many women with a history of caesarean complain of these symptoms in late pregnancy or during labour without any problems with the scar being found.

> "Women who have written to us were sectioned because their physicians were convinced that their incisions had ruptured, only to find a perfectly healthy uterus going about its business safely and efficiently."
> — **Cohen and Estner**[14]

Almost the only sign of true uterine rupture on which researchers and obstetricians agree is changes to the baby's heartbeat. However this may not be the earliest warning of problems (see Mary Cronk's views in Considering How the Baby Should Best be Monitored page 37). Many women opt for frequent hand-held monitoring together with their own pulse being monitored regularly rather than risking being made immobile with an electronic belt type monitor.

If you experience any problems relating to caesarean scar separation a caesarean can be carried out in the same way as it would be for many other emergencies.

> "Treatment of rupture of a lower segment scar does not require extraordinary facilities. Hospitals whose capabilities are so limited that they cannot deal promptly with problems associated with planning a vaginal birth after caesarean are also incapable of dealing appropriately with other obstetric emergencies. Any obstetrical department that is prepared to look after women with much more frequently

encountered conditions, such as placenta praevia, abruptio placentae, prolapsed cord, and acute fetal distress, should be able to manage a planned vaginal birth safely after a previous lower segment caesarean section."

— **Enkin et al**[3]

What Are My Chances of Having a VBAC?

This is a common question and one that can be very difficult to answer, as each woman's circumstances and personal situation will be different. Let's start with the most pessimistic figure and work up!

In the UK, just 33% of women pregnant following a caesarean section will give birth vaginally.[11] This figure is so low because many women with a history of caesarean will not even be offered the opportunity to give birth vaginally, and a substantial number will not want to.

It is impossible to state an exact VBAC rate since different research studies have used different parameters. Studies vary greatly in their decisions about which women should be advised to have a 'trial of labour' and which should not; and also the conditions under which the women laboured differed greatly. About 80% of all women who labour following a caesarean will have a VBAC.[3]

Studies also show different VBAC rates depending on the reason for the previous caesarean. Women whose caesarean was for 'failure to progress' or because the baby was believed to be in distress, have the lowest VBAC rates of around 60% upwards; whereas those who had a caesarean for breech presentation generally have VBAC rates of around 85% or more.

These differences in rates may not be caused by physical problems, but by psychological factors. Those women who had a caesarean due to breech presentation, who find their next baby is head down at the end of the following pregnancy, are already past their 'sticking point' and can confidently move into new territory. But those women who had a caesarean for 'failure to progress' or fetal distress at 9cm dilation may not believe in their ability to birth their babies until well into the labour and this might affect their ability to labour or the choices and decisions they make in labour, particularly if their caregivers are not enthusiastic about their chances of VBAC.

Despite the different figures from different research studies *The Guide to Effective Care in Pregnancy and Childbirth* has concludes that:

> "The likelihood of vaginal birth is not significantly altered by the indication for the first caesarean section (including 'cephalopelvic disproportion' and 'failure to progress'), nor by a history of more than one previous caesarean section."
>
> – Enkin et al[3]

What is clear is that women who have already had a vaginal birth either before, or following their caesarean, have much the best chance of having a VBAC.

The good news is that women who 'self-select', that is, who make their own decision that a VBAC is right for them, have the highest VBAC rates of around 90+%.[14, 15]

There is a lot you can do to increase your chances of giving birth to your baby the way you want to (see You May Have Heard You Can't Have a VBAC When..., page 18, and Making VBAC More Likely, page 24).

Research and me

You might be someone who gains an enormous amount of empowerment by reading the research on VBAC. Useful links and publications are shown at the back of this book, see also VBAC Research page 74. It is worth noting that whilst there are some immensely encouraging studies on VBAC others are less so.

Quite often we are just not able to compare like for like as different studies will be looking at different labour scenarios. Some studies don't differentiate between women who have a very medicalised 'trial of labour' with time limits and drugs being used to induce or accelerate the labour, and those who are free to labour under more conducive conditions.

"In the end I decided to stop reading the research. It was driving me mad – I was elated one minute, despondent the next as I went from one study to another. What it didn't, couldn't tell me was how likely was I to have a problem with my baby in my circumstances. I decided to rely on my gut instinct and to trust my body."

– **Elaine, VBA2C**

Comparing VBAC With Elective Repeat Caesarean

Repeat caesarean is often presented to the woman as an unselfish choice for her to make because some may think it is less risky for the baby. We live in a society which usually views any vaginal birth as risky, dangerous, and in need of a high level of medical supervision.

The research evidence on the safety of VBAC versus elective caesarean for the baby takes us into uncertain waters. As previously explained, research rarely considers longer-term outcomes, focusing mainly on the immediate effects of the birth itself and any events in the following few days spent in hospital. Even so, some studies show better outcomes for babies born by VBAC, with caesarean babies at risk of breathing problems, bruising and cuts from the operation.

> "My obstetricians told me that I would almost certainly rupture, and kill my baby if I insisted on VBACing, after all he said "the only important thing is a healthy baby" – what mother can argue with that? However as a result of the caesarean section she suffered complications and was in NICU [Neonatal Intensive Care Unit] for two weeks, the anaesthetist had great difficulty getting the spinal [anaesthetic] in and my cord was damaged resulting in long term back pain, and there was nerve damage from the incision and I have lost sensation on my stomach."
>
> – **Jo, mother of three**

If you had a 'failure to progress' labour ending in emergency section or another birth experience which has left you lacking confidence in how your body works, then repeat caesarean might seem tempting.

Women may be encouraged not to put themselves through it again. They may be told they are putting their babies at risk and setting themselves up for another failure. Perhaps this goes some way to explaining why our high national caesarean rate is made up of a large number of 'elective' repeat caesareans.

Yet how much of an informed choice is a choice made purely out of fear of the alternatives and lack of good information on the real options? Do women choose repeat caesarean because their only experience of labour is about pain and disappointment and feeling that their body let them down? Or, perhaps worse, do they choose caesarean because they cannot face trusting their bodies and their babies to health professionals who, they feel, let them down last time?

If you are caught in a dilemma of not wanting another caesarean but not wanting a difficult labour or vaginal birth either, another pregnancy may seem daunting. If you are pregnant and feeling fearful of what may happen, planning carefully can enable you to regain the confidence and control that you may have lost last time.

> "Once again, it bears mentioning that there are no published studies looking specifically at complication rates in completely unmedicated, 'natural' VBACs vs. elective repeat caesarean or a medically managed VBAC."
>
> **– Gretchen, VBAC mother and campaigner**

The decision on how to birth a next baby is rarely made on figures but on gut instinct. Indeed, most decisions made in life are not achieved after careful analysis of risks and benefits. For example, how many of us choose our means of transport based on safety statistics alone?

It may help you to focus on the fact that the risks of VBAC are small and that research only looks at trends and general outcomes. Your decision will be a personal one for this pregnancy, this baby, this time for you. VBAC can seem out of reach with too many barriers to overcome, however a good experience of VBAC is possible for most women. With good information it should be possible to plan for a vaginal birth with confidence. It might also help to try to tip the odds in your favour towards achieving your VBAC – see Making VBAC More Likely, page 24. First of all though, consider some of the barriers you may encounter.

You May Have Heard That You Can't Have a VBAC When...

Sometimes women are frightened into a repeat caesarean because they are told that something about this pregnancy makes a rupture or a repeat caesarean more likely. Common 'reasons' you may be given for not having a VBAC include:

Your previous caesarean was for 'failure to progress'/ fetal distress/a small pelvis

If your caesarean was due to 'failure to progress' at the required rate, or because the baby was thought to be in distress, you may have the impression that your body is not capable of giving birth. You may be left with doubts about whether your pelvis is big enough or the 'right' shape, or whether your uterus is capable of contracting 'properly' and efficiently.

Diseases such as rickets, which led to poorly formed bone structures, are now rare so true CPD (cephalopelvic disproportion, pelvis too small for the baby) is very uncommon in developed countries today. Although you may feel that your body failed you last time, many women come to understand that the true problem was lack of appropriate support and conditions for their labour.

Labouring in an unfamiliar environment with only strangers to care for you is known to slow labour down, make it more painful and therefore lead to more intervention for some women. When a labour is longer than average, midwives and doctors are often unable to provide appropriate support and instead offer drugs and other interventions. Sometimes a baby that is not in a very good position for labour or birth may turn with time and the right support; interventions tend to make this less likely. A long, slow labour is not in itself harmful to a healthy mother or baby, and providing both are coping well, the artificial time limits imposed by many hospitals are not helpful.

> "With Ben I'd been in hospital and things had been moved along more swiftly. If I'd been in hospital this time I'm sure that would have happened again. If I'd survived without a ruptured uterus(!) I may have been very thankful that my labour hadn't been so protracted. But with the benefit of hindsight, I am so very, very happy that

Simon was born at home. That triumph, that amazing feeling of power, that you did it by yourself, cannot be beaten."

– Tikki, after 2nd VBAC

Women can and do have successful VBACs following caesareans for 'failure to progress' and/or fetal distress, even when there is doubt over their pelvic size. Even women who have 'failed to progress' more than once have shown they are perfectly capable of giving birth vaginally in the right conditions. Many also do so with bigger babies than those for whom the caesarean was performed.[14, 16]

Your baby is too big

A 'big' baby seems to be a common worry in our society in any pregnancy, however there is no evidence that women produce babies too big for their pelvises or that big babies are more difficult to birth, particularly when women are not confined to their backs on beds.

There are no accurate methods for estimating the size of the baby, including predictions made using ultrasound and abdominal palpation (using hands to feel the baby through the abdomen).[11] A recent study showed that women themselves were almost as accurate as ultrasound at estimating the weight (especially if this wasn't their first baby) but neither were particularly accurate – ultrasound proved to be between 8 and 15% 'out'.[17]

You might, therefore, want to consider very carefully any offer of ultrasound to determine your baby's weight. If a baby actually weighs 9 pounds, a 15% error can show an ultrasound weight of 7.6 pounds (15% too low) or 10.3 pounds (15% too high)! Cases have occurred where the estimate has been as much as 2 pounds (or more than 25%) over or under actual birth weight; with a baby predicted to be 5 pounds actually weighing 7 pounds, and another predicted to be 10 pounds weighing 8 pounds.

There are several areas of concern when a baby is thought to be larger than normal. One of the more serious (but rare) is the risk of shoulder dystocia, where the baby's shoulders become stuck in the birth canal after the head has been born. However, almost half of the cases of shoulder dystocia occur in babies weighing less than 4,000g (4kg, about 8lb 12oz).[3] It has been suggested that good care from skilled birth attendants is the best way to tackle this problem, rather than resorting to an elective caesarean section 'just in case'.[3]

It is generally presumed that 'failure to progress' with a large baby means that the baby was too big for the mother. Many women, midwives and some doctors, who are more informed about natural, active birth, take the view that a larger baby simply means the labour may be longer, slower and possibly more gentle, to allow the birth to happen without causing damage to the mother.

When a baby is larger than normal it can be more important for the woman to be able to listen to her body, to be able to move freely in labour, and to adopt positions that feel right for her. Lying on her back or sitting during labour and birth can greatly reduce a woman's pelvic size.[18] Upright positions and freedom of movement make the birth easier even when the baby is smaller.

There are some encouraging 'big baby' birth stories on the homebirthuk website (see Online Resources page 83 for details).

You have had more than one previous caesarean

It seems to be a common assumption that the 'risks' of VBAC increase with the number of caesareans a woman has had. However studies have confirmed that there appears to be little, if any, difference in outcomes between women who have had one and those who have had two, three or more caesareans.

> "Obstetricians should remember that to allow a patient to labour is not a treatment, it is a virtually unavoidable consequence of pregnancy. If we are to perform a surgical procedure in order to circumvent labour we should have a clear indication. The historical evidence does not provide one and current publications indicate that we do not appear to benefit our patients by delivering them electively by caesarean section."
> — **Lawrence J. Roberts, Senior Specialist in Obstetrics and Gynaecology**[19]

There is also the assumption that having failed to give birth vaginally more than once, that the woman is unable to do so. This is rarely the case and often women who have had two or more caesareans find it helpful to assess their own needs and negotiate the type of care and conditions they require to avoid another caesarean.

Women can, and do, experience problem-free labours and give birth vaginally to healthy babies following two, three or more caesarean sections. Some choose to do so at home, sometimes attended by independent midwives, who can give the continuity and support these women may have lacked previously (see page 28 for details).

Your baby is in the breech position

Very few breech babies are born vaginally today. According to *The Sentinel Caesarean Section Audit* report the caesarean section rate for breech presentation is 88%.[11] Since the *Term Breech Trial*[20] results showing improved outcomes for breech babies born by elective caesarean section, few hospitals or obstetricians have continued their support of vaginal breech birth.

This Trial, which has convinced so may doctors that vaginal breech birth is unsafe, has been widely criticised. It did not distinguish between natural active breech birth and highly managed breech extraction (for further information see VBAC Research page 74).

ECV (external cephalic version) where the baby is turned to a head down position is often recommended to avoid breech position and consequent caesarean section. However, many doctors are reluctant to carry out this procedure on a woman with a uterine scar due to concerns that the procedure may cause the scar to separate.

Some women have opted to give birth vaginally to their breech-presenting babies and have done so without problems. Many feel, however, that the safety of vaginal breech birth is dependent on the support of a competent and confident midwife or doctor. Although there are still some practitioners within the NHS who retain the particular skills needed to assist in vaginal breech birth, they are more readily found amongst independent midwives (see page 86 for contact details).

If you are planning to labour in a hospital that routinely advises caesarean section for all women with multiple or breech babies you may face quite a lot of hostility to your VBAC plans.

This doesn't mean you are being unreasonable but it does mean you may need some skilled and confident midwifery support. Some women have found the support they need by changing their consultant or hospital.

You are carrying twins or triplets

As with breech presentation a high proportion of twin pregnancies are delivered by caesarean section (59%),[11] despite lack of evidence showing benefit for normal twin pregnancies. This is also the case for most triplets.

The additional concern in twin pregnancies following caesarean section is the possibility of extra strain on the scar. There is insufficient evidence to support this theory and some women with a history of caesarean section have given birth vaginally to healthy twins without encountering problems.[21]

It's too soon after your caesarean

Contrary to common belief, a short gap between pregnancies should not rule out a vaginal birth. Although one authority claims that a healing wound will be almost fully healed within a few weeks of a caesarean section,[22] more recent research has shown that the uterine scar does become stronger over time.

Studies have looked at women who had gaps of 6, 12, 18 and 24 months between pregnancies and the likelihood of rupture decreased very slightly with the longer the gaps.[23, 24, 25]

However the risks are small in all cases and it is perhaps more important to look at yourself and how recovered you are, both emotionally and physically. If you can, and you want to plan a longer gap, it may increase your chances of a VBAC a little but if you are pregnant again within a short time of your caesarean there is no reason to panic and it does not mean you cannot have a VBAC. Many women have healthy VBAC babies within a year of their caesarean.

Your scar is not a lower segment horizontal scar

Whilst some studies have shown increased rates of rupture for women with classical (vertical) or unusual or unknown shaped scars there are other more reassuring studies too. It seems probable that the risks are higher but still small.

> "In 1968 in Kenya, Wendy Savage delivered a woman by caesarean of her thirteenth child which was too large to pass through her pelvis. In 1946 and 1947 her first two children had been born by caesarean and she then had ten normal deliveries. During the third operation the scar of the first could hardly be seen. This incident made Wendy Savage question the inherent weakness of these scars."
>
> – **Francome et al**[26]

Women can, and do, decide to try VBAC with scars other than the usual LSCS incision.

> "The main reason I could never be allowed to labour seemed to be my previous caesarean scar, performed to save the life of my premature son. The skin incision was a horizontal 'bikini' line. Beneath this, the uterine scar was made vertically – a 'low vertical'. However, my son was born 12 weeks early, before the lower segment of the uterus had formed. Therefore, the scar was more centrally placed – a 'classical'."

Following a straightforward vaginal birth, this woman goes on to say:

> "I was never ecstatic, but the calmness I felt continued over the next few weeks. My efforts had not been wasted and there were so many advantages as well. I began to feel proud of myself and my family."
>
> – **Jacqueline, VBAC with a 'classical' incision**[27]

You are too old, too fat etc

There are a whole host of other reasons why women might be advised to have another caesarean. As we have seen above there is very little useful evidence on which to rule out VBAC. What you may find more useful is to ask your carers what their advice is based on and whether vaginal birth has additional or specific risks for you as an individual.

For example, older mothers are known to be more likely to have a caesarean birth, but that depends greatly on individual circumstances, levels of fitness, health, motivation, support, etc, just as it does for younger mothers.

If you are classed as 'high risk' and are having difficulty working out whether your individual circumstances do mean that a caesarean is advisable it might be worthwhile talking to an independent midwife.

> "No-one in their right minds should have wanted to take me on – I was 40, morbidly obese, hypertensive and with three previous caesareans – one of those for suspected pre-eclampsia. Mary didn't bat an eyelid, just said we would keep an eye on how I was and how pregnancy progressed."
>
> – Jenny, HWBA3C

Making VBAC More Likely

There are a number of things that any woman interested in having a VBAC can do to help herself. Generally these involve going over the sometimes difficult memories of you last birth experience(s) and considering what you might have done differently, as well as thinking ahead to the next birth, gathering good support and information and being clear in your mind what you really want. Consider the following points:

Thinking about previous birth experiences

If you have had a previous pregnancy end with caesarean section then you might find it hard to trust your body and you may be worried about whether you would cope or whether you would know what to do in labour. Sometimes it helps to get copies of your previous birth notes and go through them with a knowledgeable and sympathetic person who could help you work out what happened and why.

Both AIMS and NCT produce information on how to go about getting copies of your labour and delivery notes. You have a legal right to copies of notes for any baby born after 1 November 1991 (see Further Support and Information, page 85 for contact details).

"Once I understood how labour was supposed to work and how the system had failed me I got very angry. How dare they call me a failure? My body did what it should do in a stressful situation, it stopped labour, it waited for a safe, secure space in which labour could be normal. Instead of giving me that safe space, that support, they just gave me more and more drugs, more intrusions. It wasn't my failure to progress, it was their failure to support."

– Elaine, VBA2C

Some women find counselling or hypnotherapy helpful, others need to talk to people who have had similar experiences and understand how it feels. See page 84 for more information on where to find those people.

Finding support for VBAC

"Women do not refuse a 'trial of labour' when care givers truly encourage them."

– Henci Goer, Childbirth Educator and Doula[4]

The risk of the caesarean scar opening up during labour seems to loom very large in the minds of some health professionals. It is difficult to understand why this particular risk, which has been shown to be very small, should attract such attention. There are other adverse events that can happen during any pregnancy and birth which occur at least as often, but which are not highlighted in the same way, many of which are rarely discussed.

"... the probability of requiring an emergency caesarean section for acute other conditions (fetal distress, cord prolapse, or antepartum haemorrhage) in any woman giving birth, is approximately 2.7% , or up to 30 times as high as the risk of uterine rupture with a planned vaginal birth after caesarean."

– Enkin et al[3]

If you can find a caregiver who views VBAC positively, then you might feel more able to relax and give birth. It can be helpful to do your homework and find out what the attitude is to VBAC at your local maternity units. If there are several near you then you might want to go and look at them. It may be possible to find out what their caesarean and VBAC rates are. You can research this by asking the hospital or you could look at the BirthChoiceUK website (see page 83 for details). Not all hospitals will know their VBAC rate, which is disappointing, but they should be able to tell you what their elective and emergency caesarean rates are.

Many maternity units produce written 'protocols'. These are policies that the midwives and doctors should follow, however there is no reciprocal duty on your part to follow them. There may be a VBAC protocol (it might be called a 'trial of labour' protocol), which you can ask to see. This can give you valuable insight into how your prospective carers view VBAC.

> "I toured all three maternity units in my area and asked the supervisor of midwives how VBAC women were cared for, what procedures they would follow. It was really interesting to see the difference in attitudes. One talked repeatedly of scar rupture, of monitoring, not 'allowing' me to do this or 'letting' me do that. I found it helped to think of myself as the customer and that I was interviewing these people as my employees. I decided not to employ the services of people who thought so little of my chances of birthing my baby myself and who thought they had the power to 'let' or 'allow' me to do things."
>
> **– Elaine, VBA2C**

Some women are told at their booking in appointment that they are 'high risk' because of their previous caesarean and will have to see the consultant and have to have consultant led or shared care. This is not the case. You have the same care options as, and rights of, any other pregnant woman.

The AIMS book *Am I Allowed?* gives comprehensive details of your rights in pregnancy and birth. You are not obliged to see anyone if you don't want to, nor can you be forced to do something or accept treatment you don't feel is right (see page 78 for details).

You may choose to meet your named obstetrician as you may decide that it would be useful to see what his or her attitude is on VBAC. You might be surprised – he or she may be very happy with the idea and be keen to support you. However, if they are neutral or hostile to VBAC and keen to tell you only about the risks and scare you into a repeat caesarean, this can be quite a difficult appointment. It might help to take another person with you as well as your partner, particularly if your partner is unsure about, or hostile to, the idea of VBAC. You also have the right to get up and leave at any time.

Many of us have been brought up to believe that doctor knows best and it can be very hard to feel you have to argue your case with someone who you think is better informed and trained than yourself. Sometimes we feel the need for the approval of our caregivers for our plans, and can feel devastated when this approval is withheld or is muted. Some women go very deeply into the research evidence and go armed with facts and figures prepared for an argument or some hard negotiation. Some go with the attitude of not caring what is said – they know what they want. Some don't go at all.

> "I took the advice of various friends, including a midwife, not to enter into any dialogue with hospital consultants. I could not change their attitudes, and it was not worth the risk of me being undermined and upset."
>
> **– Caroline, VBAC**

Your carers have an obligation to ensure that they have given you the opportunity to make an informed choice. If you decline an opportunity to discuss VBAC with an obstetrician it should merely be noted, no one should try to make you attend. If you feel confident and assertive you could go and interview your obstetrician with a view to leaving if you are feeling undermined or under attack. You can choose to be cared for by another obstetrician or to opt for midwife only care.

Medical professionals, like their clients, have differing views on birth, VBAC and caesareans. If it is important to you to get a 'seal of approval' for your VBAC plans then you might have to do quite a bit of searching or you might find that your local midwives and obstetricians are very open and receptive to your plans. It can be helpful to contact the Supervisor of Midwives at the hospital, to seek her help in finding a supportive obstetrician and/or midwives.

You could pay for a private consultation if you can find an obstetrician who is supportive of VBAC. You don't have to go on and book with that obstetrician, just getting an opinion that you know won't be automatically hostile might be important to you. Above all, you might want to ask yourself what outcome are you looking for, what information do you need, is it important to you to seek 'approval' from someone medically qualified and if so why?

If you are finding it difficult to find support you may wish to seek help from AIMS or from some of the other sources on pages 85.

Finding good midwifery support

> "I didn't want or need anyone's approval to have this baby vaginally. I knew deep down in my gut that I could do it. But I knew I needed a wise woman."
>
> – Jenny, HWBA3C

Midwives are the experts in normal birth. The quality and quantity of midwifery care makes a difference to birth outcomes. Having someone who supports your plans and knows how to help you achieve them, whilst being trained to look out for the abnormal, should make a difference to your labour. When women are not relaxed, not happy with their carers or their environment, they are more likely to labour longer or not labour at all. If you translate this to a VBAC labour where the woman might have a previous poor experience of labour, how much more important is it that she should have someone with her whom she trusts?

For some women it might not be important, they might have the confidence to block out any perceived tension or fear or hostility from their midwives. For others it might be the crucial factor in their being able to achieve a VBAC.

> "My NHS midwife was fantastic, an advocate for me and thoroughly supportive throughout...she restored my faith in my body and inspired me so much that I am training to be a midwife myself. She changed my perspective of birth and I realised that I could be a 'Woman' and do it myself! I thought birth was like an appointment until my second pregnancy and the result was a huge belief in myself and feelings of euphoria. I believed I could do anything!"
>
> – Lin, VBAC

Maternity units vary all over the country in how they organise their staff. Some will have small teams of midwives who operate a 'caseload' which means that you should get to know everyone in your team and you are much more likely to have someone with you in labour that you know. However in many areas this doesn't happen and you may be attended in labour by strangers.

This might not be a problem to you. For some women the presence of a known midwife is incidental to their labour. However for many, the midwife is the person they look to for support in labour. If your previous experience of labour was difficult, or you have never laboured before, knowing your midwife might be really important to you. Also, being in control, including having control over who is with you when you are at your most vulnerable, may be very important, particularly for those who had an unhappy labour previously.

> "I knew the day that Toby was born that I was going to have an independent midwife next time around. I organised my care before I was pregnant. It was wonderful to be in control, I had no scans, no visits to hospital or doctors and no tests, other than a few blood tests. I felt it was important for me not to treat this pregnancy as a medical event. I was able to spend hours talking about my pregnancy, previous births and my hopes and concerns for this birth"
>
> – Debbie, VBA3C

So how do you get the midwifery care you want and need? Firstly, you can find out what is on offer, perhaps by talking to other local women and/or talking to your local community midwife. AIMS or NCT may be able to put you in contact with people who know about your local maternity services (see page 84 for contact details). If you have more than one maternity unit to choose from you can try talking to the Supervisor of Midwives at each one.

An appointment with the Supervisor of Midwives can also provide an opportunity to discuss your circumstances, explain that you are keen to achieve a normal birth, and ask what level of midwifery support you can expect. It is often worth asking if you can be assigned to the care of a midwife or midwives who are comfortable with VBAC labour and who will be supportive of what you wish to achieve.

One way of increasing your chances of having a midwife you know is to book a home birth. Although this does not guarantee that a midwife you have met will attend you in labour, in many instances this will be the case. However, for those who do not feel comfortable with the idea of a homebirth, suggesting it may be the leverage that gets you the care you want.

> "Having been told that I must go into hospital and be monitored continuously and that I wasn't allowed to use the birthing pool and I had to give birth within a certain time limit, I decided to have a home birth. I didn't think their plans for my VBAC would help me to labour. When I told my midwife she didn't say much but soon I got a phone call from the Supervisor of Midwives. Suddenly I could use the home-from-home room, use the birthing pool, have a midwife come out and assess me at home and accompany me into hospital. Anything seemed possible if I would only give up my home birth plan which they seemed to find terrifying."
> — **Elaine VBA2C**

Where women are unable to find the midwifery support they are looking for, they may look outside the NHS for their maternity care. An independent midwife might seem like an impossible luxury but most are able to accept fees in instalments, some over a long period, making it more accessible. Some couples re-mortgage or take out a loan to pay the fees, others might enter into a bartering arrangement if the midwife is agreeable and they have skills she needs. It is usual to have an initial interview with your prospective midwife to explore compatibility and options before any commitment is made.

> "When you approach a VBAC, it feels a bit as if you are being set up as a failure from the outset. It's refreshing to have someone look after you, who gives you back the confidence you are so sadly lacking when faced with the constant barrage of 'risks' and 'complications'. I had to employ independent midwives to achieve this."
> — **Tikki, HBA2C**

Considering other birth supporters

Some women have found it immensely reassuring and helpful to employ a doula. A doula is a trained and paid supporter who can provide support during labour, birth, and/or the postnatal period. She cannot give medical care but she can help you and your partner at the birth (and beyond in some instances). Her role is to support your decisions and support you and your partner emotionally – perhaps helping you move into comfortable positions, massaging and encouraging you (see pages 84 and 86 for contact details).

You might also consider having the support of other birth companions such as a friend or a relative, in addition to your partner. This should ideally be someone who believes in your ability to give birth and who is not going to be frightened or anxious about your VBAC. Fear and anxiety are easily communicated to a labouring woman, often by non-verbal means, and this could have an effect on your labour. Women who have had a positive experience of birth themselves can be particularly helpful in this role.

> "Your best chance of a normal birth is to have a spontaneous, uninterfered-with labour surrounded by people you know and trust in an environment most conducive to that."
>
> – **Rosie, Midwife**

Considering a home birth

We live in a society that thinks it knows that birth is dangerous and so home birth must be doubly dangerous. Add a VBAC into that equation and you are likely to face some incredulity. Reading the evidence on home birth can be a real eye-opener.

> "I thought I was well informed. I'd read loads of books and magazines, I had a bit of nursing experience. I thought that women who home birthed were lentil eating madwomen who carelessly put their babies' lives in danger. I wanted to be where the medical equipment was. Two caesareans later, I read the evidence and realised where 'being where the medical equipment was' had got me."
>
> – **Jenny, HBA3C**

There is plenty of evidence now on general home birth safety; there is less on home birth after caesarean although a study on home birth in 1997 showed a 72% success rate in women in the home birth group who had had a previous caesarean with no reported adverse outcomes attributed to HBAC.[28] Yet the attraction of homebirth is not just about relative safety in terms of birth outcomes. For many women it's about emotional and psychological safety, it's also about being empowered and taking control of their labours. Some women just cannot face another hospital experience and feel instinctively that they would not labour well, if at all, in hospital because of their anxiety.

> "My husband and I wanted to give birth at home. A decision we were both happy with. I didn't trust hospitals or their policy on VBAC. I didn't feel that 'their way' was safe and all I wanted was a safe birth!!! I didn't want to feel threatened or intimidated. I wanted to feel in control."
>
> – **Edita, VBAC**

There is some good physiology behind those instinctive feelings. We know that women who are anxious don't labour well; in fact their bodies can slow or stop labour until they are in a relaxed state.

The Birthday Trust report[28] which looked at home birth in general found that women who planned a home birth halved their risk of caesarean, forceps and ventouse delivery, were less likely to have a postpartum haemorrhage, had fewer episiotomies and were less likely to use drugs for pain relief. The benefits weren't confined to the women either; the babies had better APGAR scores and were more likely to breastfeed.

We don't know how many of the benefits of home birth can be translated into benefits for the VBAC woman because the research has not been carried out. However if you ask independent midwives what their experiences and statistics are on home birth after caesarean, they report good outcomes.

You have a right to give birth at home. There are Trusts that are reluctant to provide a midwife for a home birth, particularly where a woman has a caesarean scar. For further information on midwifery provision for home births see *Am I Allowed?* (details on page 78).

Many women opt out of hospital birth because they feel that a home birth gives them a greater chance of achieving a successful VBAC. It is unfortunate that so many women are not given the opportunity to labour in hospital with the individual support of a midwife and without the constant pressure of time limits and continuous electronic fetal monitoring.

Considering a birth centre or midwife-led unit

If home birth feels a step too far then trying to find a maternity unit with a low tech or 'home-from-home' room might be an option to explore.

Sadly, some birthing centres or midwife-led units have policies which classify you as 'high risk' and they are not able to accept your booking. This seems inappropriate, as VBAC women need the same care and equipment as any other women having a vaginal birth. According to its website, the Birth Centre in Tooting has had a VBAC rate of 95% in recent years, which is a much higher figure than most hospitals can claim. Sometimes though it is possible to negotiate, so you might want to consider contacting the Head of Midwifery at the unit.

Considering induction

If your pregnancy continues much beyond your estimated due date this can leave you in a bit of a dilemma. You might be told that if you go a certain number of days over 40 weeks and your unit does not offer induction to VBAC women, your only option is elective, repeat caesarean.

> "I was 'allowed' to go ten days over but was then cut, after threats of 'dead baby, dead mother'. Failure to wait. Failure to fight. Failure to know better. I was told he would be very big. He weighed 9lbs 1 oz."
> – **Rach, VBA2C** (her VBAC baby weighed 10lbs 2oz; see also Jenna's birth story, page 46)

Some units now have a policy of no induction for women who have had a previous caesarean. There are concerns that prostaglandin gel pessaries (a common way of starting labour off), could have an adverse affect on caesarean scar tissue. Research evidence suggests that prostaglandin gel pessaries might increase the risk of uterine rupture by about 4 times, to a level of around 24 per 1,000.[29]

There are even greater concerns over a particular prostaglandin, misoprostol, which is not licensed for obstetric use in this country, and which have prompted NICE (the National Institute for Clinical Excellence) to recommend that its use be confined to clinical trials.[30]

Although many hospitals do not routinely induce women with a uterine scar, some obstetricians are of the opinion that although there is an increased risk with induction, it is still an option to consider; for example where the alternative is an immediate caesarean, such as in some cases of pre-eclampsia.

As with many other decisions, it is a case of balancing the risks and benefits, and individual circumstances can tip the balance in favour of induction under carefully monitored conditions. Providing that those caring for the woman are aware of the risks and warning signs and that recourse to a caesarean in the event of a suspected rupture can be prompt, then any additional risk to the mother or baby may be small, and possibly less than that of going straight to an elective caesarean.

But just how much of a problem is going past your estimated due date? Our society does seem to have a strong belief that placentas have a shelf life or a use by date and that 40 weeks is full term. The World Health Organization defines normal pregnancy as between 37 and 42 weeks. Different methods of calculating a due date can also give dates which are several days apart.

The length of a woman's menstrual cycle can make a difference, as women with longer cycles will have conceived later and will therefore tend to have longer pregnancies.

Lengths of pregnancies do vary. It is well documented that there are differences between ethnic groups in terms of average lengths of pregnancies and women who have a longer pregnancy often comment that others in their family have experienced this too. It may be worth considering whether a longer pregnancy is just normal for the genetic makeup of your babies.

> "My husband was born at 44 weeks and his brother at 43 weeks, so I could clearly place the blame on our children's reluctance to be born on their father!"
> – **Debbie, HWBA3Cs**

There is evidence that reducing the number of women who go over 42 weeks reduces the number of stillbirths but the numbers are very small. Often women are told that the risk of stillbirth 'doubles', but if you look at the actual research figures on which this is based the rate increases from 1 per 3,000 at 37 weeks to 3 in 3000 at 42 weeks to 6 in 3000 at 43 weeks.[30] There is also a similar increase in baby deaths around the time of birth. So while the risk increases, it remains low.

Despite the NICE recommendation that women with uncomplicated pregnancies should be "offered" induction beyond 41 weeks, there have not been sufficiently large trials comparing continuing a pregnancy with induction of labour, to enable the effects on stillbirth rates to be fully assessed.

The reasoning behind the recommendation is that as a 43-week pregnancy has a higher stillbirth rate, by reducing the length of the pregnancy you will reduce the risk of stillbirth to the same level of that of pregnancies that naturally end at 42 weeks. There is no evidence currently that this strategy is actually effective.

Apart from induction or an elective caesarean you do have a third option. You can opt to wait for an 'overdue' labour to start spontaneously with or without increased monitoring and checks on you and the baby. The NICE guideline practice recommendation for those who decline induction or caesarean states:

> "From 42 weeks, women who decline induction of labour should be offered increased antenatal monitoring consisting of a twice weekly CTG and ultrasound estimation of maximum amniotic pool depth." [30]

You do not have to accept monitoring if you don't want to – you have the right to refuse.

If you are being advised to accept induction or repeat caesarean for other reasons then these reasons should be explained clearly to you, along with why the risks of induction or repeat caesarean in your particular case outweigh the risks of waiting for labour to start.

If you are surrounded by people who are getting very anxious about the length of your pregnancy, or if you are feeling uncertain or undermined yourself, then you might find it helpful to talk to other VBAC women who have had 'longer' pregnancies. See page 85 for contact details of sources of support and AIMS' publication *Induction - Do I Really Need It?* page 80.

Deciding when to go into hospital and how long to labour

It is common to advise a woman planning a VBAC that she 'must' come into hospital as soon as she knows she is in labour and that she 'must' have the baby within a certain time frame. This advice is based on concerns about possible problems with the scar. The risks of a caesarean scar separation are very small (see What About Caesarean Scar Rupture?' page 11), and there is no evidence that longer labours cause an increase in the risk of scar separation.

Given that we know tension and anxiety are likely to slow labour down and that many VBAC women have had poor previous experiences of hospital, early admission to hospital and time limits are quite likely to result in another caesarean because of 'failure to progress'. Women who have never laboured before, or who have had a labour which didn't proceed to second stage, are likely to labour like a first time mother. Arbitrary time limits and the medical interventions that go with them in an attempt to make us to birth our babies quickly, are not likely to be helpful.

Going to the hospital too early in labour could also mean that labour will be deemed to have started earlier, the clock will therefore start ticking earlier, and the woman will be put at an unfair additional disadvantage and be even less likely to be able to labour within the prescribed time limits.

If you are planning a hospital birth it might be worth thinking about when you want to go in. If you are in good, strong, established labour when you go into hospital you are less likely to be affected by the memories of last time, the smells, the sounds, the general distractions of admission. However, you may need to balance this with making a journey during a later stage of labour. A long and complicated journey may also be a factor to consider.

> "I went on the hospital tour of the labour ward, just to remind myself where everything was really. I'm glad I did because when I saw the labour room, unchanged since last time, I completely freaked. All the memories came rushing back and I was panic-stricken. Imagine if I had been in labour, what would that have done to my contractions?"
>
> – Elaine VBA2C

As for timing labour, many midwives will tell you that the clock is an unreliable tool in any labour. Providing that you are labouring well and the baby is showing no signs of distress, there is no evidence that the strength of your scar has some kind of time limit. Indeed a long, slow labour might be what your body needs to do.

When it comes to second stage, some hospitals will have time limits on that too. Those time limits may not take into account the pause that sometimes happens between first and second stage. Second stage may be measured from the moment the woman is found (or thought) to be fully dilated, rather than from the time that the baby begins to be spontaneously and actively pushed out by the uterus. Even then, providing mother and baby are well there is no evidence that time limits make birth safer.

> "Medical practitioners are often so stressed by what they see as the potential dangers of VBAC that many do not have the confidence to allow the mother to labour in her own time. They want the birth concluded as quickly as possible, to get to the point where the perceived spectre has passed ...If, the only reason a speedy delivery is being considered is that the sand in the egg timer has run out...there is little justification for mending what is not broken."
> – **Lowdon & Chippington Derrick**[31]

Considering how the baby should best be monitored

It is very common for hospitals to have a policy of continuous electronic fetal heart monitoring (CEFM) for VBAC women. If you haven't previously experienced this, it involves having two wide 'belts' around your abdomen with round discs called 'transducers'; one positioned towards the top of your abdomen, which 'listens' to your contractions, and the other lower down, which 'listens' to the baby's heartbeat. It produces a printed 'trace' of what the baby's heartbeat is doing with each contraction.

This might sound great in theory but in practice it can have a huge impact on your labour, as quite often you have to be still during contractions so that the monitor can pick up the baby's heartbeat accurately. For many women the monitor is very uncomfortable and restricting because it prevents them moving around and adopting upright positions which can be the most helpful way of dealing with labour pain. There is also evidence that women who are free to move about and adopt positions of their choosing will labour more quickly and with less need for medical interventions.[32]

CEFM is also known to increase the incidence of caesarean section, mainly because it identifies more babies as being in difficulty when they are not. There is no evidence that this improves the outcome for mother or baby, nor that it is necessary in a VBAC labour. CEFM has been shown to be difficult to interpret correctly and does not benefit babies or women in straightforward labour.[33]

There are alternatives to continuous monitoring. A midwife can listen to the baby's heart rate with a pinard, a wooden or plastic ear trumpet. This is usually done every 15 to 20 minutes during active labour and is likely to be at least as frequent as the trace of a continuous monitor is checked.

The midwife could also use a handheld sonicaid, which uses ultrasound in the same way as the larger belt monitor, and enables the baby's heart rate to be heard as well as giving digital rates. Alternatively the belt monitor from a CEFM can be used as a hand held monitor, allowing a printed trace to be recorded for a short period of time, perhaps with the midwife or birth partner holding it in place.

Whilst there seems to be a widespread belief amongst obstetricians that CEFM will forewarn them of a scar rupture, is there actually any evidence to support this belief?

> "In order for CEFM to be of assistance to the attending practitioner, it needs to be observed continuously or at least very frequently. If the attending practitioner is therefore in frequent or continuous attendance there is no reason why intermittent auscultation cannot be performed, and frequent observation of the woman's behaviour and demeanour, pulse rate and perhaps blood pressure.
>
> "If the rationale behind routine CEFM is that a non-reassuring trace will indicate scar compromise, I believe that fetal heart problems are a late sign of scar dehiscence. I feel that there are signs and symptoms of scar compromise that can become apparent before the baby and the baby's heart is affected. Such as: the woman's demeanour changes, she may inform her attendant that she is feeling pain

between contractions, and that the pain is different. If she has been encouraged to feel her own scar antenatally she will recognise any significant increase in tenderness. Her pulse rate will increase quite markedly from HER normal rate, which should have been recorded in her antenatal notes.

"I feel that reliance on routine CEFM can detract from the attendant's careful clinical observations and delay recognition of scar compromise. And that the presence of a reassuring trace may give a false reassurance.

"The use of CEFM does of course immobilise the woman to a greater or lesser extent and this in itself can inhibit the progress of labour and reduce the chances of a successful VBAC. The attendant's preoccupation with the fetal heart monitor and its printout may detract from the support, help, and close observation she is able to offer the labouring woman"

– **Mary Cronk, Independent Midwife**[34]

You have an absolute right to say no to any 'treatment', including monitoring, that you are offered. In fact, your carers should ask for your informed consent to this, as with any procedure. You may want to tell your carers that you don't consent to this beforehand so that you will not become anxious in labour about having to go into hospital and 'fight' over monitoring. It doesn't matter if something is hospital policy; this just means that the staff may be obliged to offer or suggest it, but they cannot impose it, and your informed refusal should just be respected.

It can be very unnerving to refuse something suggested by a medical professional and so having good, informed support around you – from partner, relatives, doula, antenatal teacher or independent midwife, etc – can be very helpful.

Using birth pools or 'home-from-home' rooms

If your hospital perceives VBAC to be a risky business then you are likely to come across problems over the use of their birthing pool, 'home-from-home' room or other comfort measures which may be restricted to 'low risk' women. Some women have found that expressing an interest home birth can result in changes of attitude, but it is probably a good idea to ensure you have any agreement reached recorded in writing on your notes.

If you are booking a home birth anyway, then choosing whether to hire a pool is your decision. Most independent midwives and some NHS midwives are quite comfortable with the idea of VBAC labours and births in water.

Some suggest that the support of the water for the labouring uterus might be positively beneficial. There is also recent research which shows that use of a water pool significantly reduces reported pain and may shorten labour.[35]

Considering the need for a cannula

Some hospitals may suggest that you have a cannula (needle) for an intravenous drip inserted into your arm or hand while in labour. The theory is that if your scar should rupture, then blood loss could make access to a vein difficult, although as already explained the likelihood of this happening is very small. Inserting a cannula earlier would allow fluids to be given and could enable a caesarean to be carried out with less delay.

Although some mothers find this nothing more than a minor inconvenience, a cannula can be irritating and painful, and may be a constant, demoralising reminder of an expectation of failure. Some women who have been willing to accept this have used it as a trade-off against other interventions. As with any intervention, your consent would be required, and you have a right to decline.

Encouraging the baby into a good position for labour ('optimal fetal positioning')

Over the last decade there has been increasing interest from mothers and midwives about 'optimal fetal positioning'.[36] It literally means: optimal = best; fetal = baby; positioning = position in the uterus. Optimal fetal positioning is about how the position of the baby in late pregnancy and early labour might affect the labour itself (see Further Reading page 78 for details of *Understanding and Teaching Optimal Foetal Positioning* by Jean Sutton and Pauline Scott, and *Sit Up and Take Notice* by Pauline Scott).

Babies who lie in a posterior position in the uterus; that is with the baby's backbone lying towards your back, often seem to go past their estimated due date and may result in a long, slow, backache labour. It is thought the contractions try to move the baby to a better position before second stage.

In the final months of pregnancy it can help to use positions which will encourage the baby to move round into an anterior position, that is with the baby's back facing into your front, preferably towards the left hand side.

Spending time on hands and knees or kneeling up and leaning into a pile of cushions, a beanbag or rocking on a birthing ball may help. Positions that generally work best are those that are upright and/or leaning forward where your hips are higher than your knees.

Janet Balaskas has also written about active birth and pre-pregnancy exercises to help make birth more straightforward (see the Further Reading page 78 for details).

Using upright positions for labour

Women who are unmedicated and free to move in labour often comment about how important it was for them to be able to move around freely and adopt whatever positions seemed right and most comfortable for them at the time.

Many women find that upright positions work best, enabling them to lean forward in labour and to rock or sway. This not only helps women deal with the pain of contractions, it also helps the labour to progress smoothly.

Research supports this theory, showing that this instinctive behaviour makes good sense as it not only reduces the pain, it makes labour shorter and less likely to need medical interventions.[32]

> "Like a long distance runner, you just find your rhythm. I found a position perched on the edge of the bed which really worked for me. I kept mobile, kept upright."
> – **Rach, VBA2C**

See the Further Reading section on page 78 for more information on positions for labour and birth, and the AIMS publication *Birthing Your Baby – The Second Stage*. Some antenatal classes might also be helpful.

Thinking about pain relief

A common concern among women planning a VBAC is how they will cope with the pain of labour. This worry is particularly common among women who had an elective caesarean and have therefore not laboured before.

In the majority of cases, women who are able to maintain a level of control with which they are comfortable, who have good support from their birth companions, and who are free to move and adopt positions they find most comfortable, find they are able to cope well with labour and that they experience far less pain.

> "My midwife showed me where the gas and air was; I knew it was there when the pain got worse. However, I was so busy labouring and giving birth, that I actually forgot all about it."
>
> – Debbie, HWBA3Cs

If you do feel you would like some pain relief to help you through, all the usual options should be available to you. Although there is some concern that using an epidural in a VBAC labour may mask signs of scar rupture, this doesn't seem to be borne out by any research and certainly many obstetricians don't discourage epidural use.

However, an epidural is much more likely to put you in an immobile position with all the disadvantages that can bring and may make a ventouse or forceps or even a repeat caesarean more likely.

For further information see Further Reading page 78 for details of *Birthing from Within* by Pam England and Rob Horowitz, and *Ina May's Guide to Childbirth*.

Planning Your VBAC

Making a decision about your birth choices after a previous caesarean birth may be something you did straight after your caesarean experience, or it might have been a long and drawn out process lasting several months. You might find that your feelings change during the course of the pregnancy. It is not unusual to suddenly feel fearful as the birth approaches and this may be a time to re-read this booklet or to contact some of the support people and services in the appendix of this book. You might not reach a final decision until you are at the end of your pregnancy, or indeed in labour.

There are some very helpful articles on planning a VBAC which are listed in the Online Resources, pages 83. Of course you cannot plan for every eventuality. In the end, a positive belief in yourself and your body and its ability to birth your healthy baby seems to shine through many of the VBAC birth stories which women have been kind enough to share.

Many women seem to find it helpful to put their own limits on the possibilities, writing birth plans or agreeing plans of care which say things like *"In the event of labour not progressing smoothly I do not consent to oxytocic drugs, forceps or ventouse, I want a repeat caesarean"*. For many women the VBAC itself is not the only or ultimate goal and you may want to think about the circumstances under which you would decide to have another caesarean.

> "There is a perception that if the woman has the responsibility, that the level of risk is somehow increased, but I believe very strongly that when the woman has responsibility safety is ensured, because a caesarean mother would never risk her baby – she will always make the sacrifice she has made in the past if she believes for one moment that it is necessary.
>
> "Women do not go against medical advice lightly and in all the years I have been working with caesarean mothers I have never come across a case of a woman who has gone against medical advice and lived to regret it. However, women do 'give in' to their concerns and transfer to the medical model of birth, and live to regret the consequences. In addition, I have heard my fair share of tragic stories, and without exception, they have been the result of poor care never the result of a woman's ill-advised decisions. Only you can give birth to your baby – other people can only deliver it for you – and there is a world of difference between the two."
>
> **– Gina, HBAC, and VBAC campaigner**

Having made a decision the important thing to many women seems to be not whether the birth was caesarean or vaginal, but how they feel about it afterwards. In other words, any way of birth is positive, if you feel positively about it. I hope this book has helped you to think about what it is that you want from this next birth and has given you some strategies to achieve the best possible birth for you in your circumstances.

> "So many times I had dreamed of this in my relaxation sessions but oh the triumph of the realisation of those dreams. I had expected to be exulted, elated but it went deeper than that. A deep quiet "Yes." An affirmation of everything I held to be true about the power of the female body and spirit. The triumph of hope over previous experience."
>
> – **Jenny, HWBA3C**

VBAC birth reports

Reading books and research may be helpful to you but some women gain enormous comfort and support from hearing about other people's VBAC experiences. Obviously, no two births will be the same but it can be very helpful to know of people who have had a VBAC. Here are just a few, with many thanks to the women who kindly volunteered to share their experiences in the hope that they might help to inspire someone else.

Theo's birth - A Vaginal Birth After a Previous Classical Incision Caesarean

My Mum had home births so when I became pregnant with my first son, Ryan, this was where I hoped to be. Unfortunately, because of a rather large fibroid right in the way of the baby, I ended up having a classical caesarean. The stay in hospital afterwards was so awful I decided that if I had another child that I would want to be at home, despite being told by my consultant that I must have another caesarean.

When, three years later, I found out I was expecting again I contacted Lynn, an independent midwife. We made plans for home birth but prepared to transfer in if we needed to. At Lynn's suggestion we met a consultant locally who is pro VBAC.

Labour started one Sunday evening. I had my first contraction but it wasn't until I'd had a few more that I realised that yes this was finally it. Things continued through the night but tailed off towards morning so we tried to continue as normal. The same thing happened later on Tuesday evening. By Wednesday I was tired and a bit despondent. That evening when having a bath I had a show and later in bed I felt my waters go. On Thursday evening Lynn came and, she told us that the baby had got himself into an awkward position. She said that some time spent on hands and knees with my bum in the air would help him turn.

The contractions had tailed off again so we went to bed hoping for some sleep. I made myself a nest of pillows trying to keep my bum as high in the air as possible. This is not the most comfortable of positions when heavily pregnant. About midnight I was awakened by the urge to go to the loo but the biggest contraction I had ever felt took over. I yelled at Simon to help me out of bed; as he did I had the urge to push!

I felt very frightened and not really sure what was happening which sounds a bit silly but I never got as far as the pushing stage last time. We made it to the bathroom where another contraction and the urge to push took hold. I was telling Simon to call Lynn. He tried to get me to talk to her but I just kept asking him to tell her to come.

Lynn finally arrived and asked if I wanted to go to hospital. I said a very definite no. With Lynn around I felt much calmer. I spent the next few hours on my knees over the bath having sips of water, squeezing Simon's hand very tightly and making the most amazing noises. Lynn was checking the baby's heartbeat and my pulse, rubbing my back and shoulders and giving me lots of encouragement.

A little later Lynn said she could see the baby's head but it kept slipping back so she encouraged me to change position. We tried a few contractions with me standing with my arms around Simon's neck but this still wasn't helping so she suggested a birthing stool. As soon as I sat down on it the baby's head immediately came down and started crowning!

Simon sat on a child's step stool behind me and slowly but surely the contractions pushed the head out. The rest of him shot out in one contraction! Lynn caught him, put him straight on to my tummy and put a towel over both of us to keep him warm. A little later, Simon held Theo and a sleepy Ryan came in to meet his new little brother, it was so nice that he could meet him so soon after the birth. Afterwards we all moved to our bedroom, it was so wonderful to be able to get into my own bed and the rest of the day was spent there. It was a very different experience from the birth of my first son.

– **Sarah Carreck**

Jenna's Birth Story – a VBA2C

It was Friday, I was 2 weeks overdue by my dates, longer by the hospital's. Every day that passed piled on the pressure. My midwives had to refer me for an appointment with the consultant which was set for Monday. I really had no idea what labour was going to be like. I had two children, but had never given birth. Never even had a contraction.

On Friday, I had a lot of Braxton Hicks. My favourite midwife rang to tell me she was on call all weekend. It all seemed almost too good to be true. I spent the night relishing this new experience: lights out, keeping moving, silent, resting on my birth ball. I kept on having strong but not painful contractions till around 3.40am. Then they stopped. I tried not to be disappointed, and got some sleep.

I was woken up by a stronger contraction at 6.30am. DH [dear husband] gave me a hug and kiss, I said "They're still going!" and his whole face lit up. The kids came bouncing in, we all got up and had breakfast together. I was starting to believe that this was it, but was surprised: I had been listening to other people's birth stories, and mine was different. I said to DH "But I haven't had a show yet!" then went to the toilet, and had a show.

We had intended to stay at home as long as possible – till at least 7cm dilated, and maybe having an "accidentally on purpose" home birth. Something told me however that I should call and just let the midwife know. She sounded almost as excited as me. I said no hurry, we were going out for a walk to the post office. It's only a five-minute walk, but I had to stop a couple of times to get through contractions. I had my TENS machine on, and was trying to keep the wires hidden so no one would work out I was in labour. The post office was really busy, and I had five contractions while trying to hide behind the birthday cards! I did get some strange looks.

My contractions weren't at all what I expected. I thought the pain would be around my scar area and cervix. Instead I felt them in my lower back and across the front of my thighs. This was a relief: at least I couldn't get worried that the pain was my old scars rupturing. I felt no pain around my scar area throughout. Each contraction was an incredibly powerful surge, a building force inside me, like thunder brewing. With each one, in these early stages, I was focusing on relaxing, thinning and opening. Kept trying to visualise those beautiful orange lilies unfolding, and hoping my cervix was doing the same. I kept telling myself that each surge was bringing my baby closer to me. Each one done was one less to be done.

Things seemed to be getting stronger, the midwife rang back and I said I'd quite like the baby checked out. About 5 minutes later I had a big contraction and my waters started to go. When I looked down, my heart sank. I really thought at this point that my VBAC was scuppered: the waters were basically brown. As soon as the midwife, Julie, came into my room I showed her the meconium. She kept her voice very steady but I could tell she was worried. The heartbeat was fine, and we all breathed a sigh of relief. Our friends were on their way to look after the children. Julie, asked that we leave as soon as they arrived. My two-year-old son was very tearful, so it was hard leaving. The journey was great, just me and DH, driving through our beautiful Welsh countryside, listening to one of the tapes he had made for me. We stopped for petrol and illicit snacks. We took our time.

When we arrived at the hospital, Julie was waiting outside for us. The delivery room was bleak. We put the music back on. Pretty soon I was assessed: 3cms dilated but 100% effaced, baby high and head transverse. At least I had started dilating. The SHO [Senior House Officer, a student doctor] who assessed me said she could feel some membranes in front of the baby's head, which she would remove. I said that I did NOT want her to remove them. I did agree however, as per my birth plan, to have a cannula inserted and had some blood taken. The SHO said she'd be back in a couple of hours.

I tried hard to get things how I wanted, to find a good position. Because of the meconium, I was strapped to monitors, but refused to lie down and kept going to the toilet – any excuse to get away from the machine that goes ping. I tried gas & air. At first I hated it. I felt a bit drunk, and I didn't want to be out of control. Five minutes later however, I was asking to try it again!

When the SHO came back, I was found to be 3-4cm, and the baby was still high. I was incredibly disappointed. The SHO asked me not to eat or drink, as I was high risk. She actually asked my DH first, when I was in the toilet, but he suggested she talk to me. I disagreed. A midwife asked me to confirm this decision, as she had to write it down. The SHO said we were not making enough progress. She would "give us" another two hours, but then we would need to "look at alternatives".

At this point I had my moment of doubt. I knew I needed to relax, I knew the contractions needed to be more effective. I knew all this, and yet I wanted an epidural. I wanted to rest. Everything I knew about epidurals didn't seem to matter. I thought things were going to get worse. It really did seem to make sense. Thank goodness for my DH and my midwife. The midwife suggested we try gas & air for a bit longer. DH said that if I had an epidural, I would not have my VBAC. When the SHO returned to ask was I waiting for an epidural, I quickly said no.

From that point on, things went much better. My waters seemed to just keep going. Each gush brought more meconium, which DH and the midwife quickly cleared away in case the doctors panicked. DH and I had lots of cuddles and kisses, we listened to our music, I asked for the blinds to be shut, started to go more within myself. During one intense contraction someone barged straight into the room. After that, I asked for a sign to be put on the door. Taking charge in small ways like this made a real difference to us. Even just wearing my own clothes was important.

The next time the SHO came in, I was 6cm. The baby was still high, but it felt like real progress. The doctors looked at the monitor output and were concerned about the heartbeat. DH and Julie told them that these were losses of contact where I had changed position. Poor Julie spent hours on her hands and knees trying to keep a good contact: there was no way I was lying down, and not moving. We never had any doubts about the baby's heartbeat but the doctors said they had to call my obstetrician.

When he came, he was unconcerned and very supportive – a far cry from his attitude antenatally. Later, he wanted to put an internal scalp monitor on. I asked whether this would stop me moving, he quickly said no. Once more onto the bed, once more writhing in agony. I was very vocal at this point! My obstetrician gave me the best news. The baby's head was now anterior and I was 7cms. The obstetrician said he thought "we were going to get away with this", that he felt the baby would come vaginally, I may need a bit of help but that was all. When questioned further he said he meant maybe forceps or ventouse. I was on cloud nine and really did not care: I knew now that I could do this.

About 9.00pm, I felt a bit pushy towards the end of each contraction. My midwife noticed and asked if she could examine me, and I was happy for her to. She said I was about 9.5cms with a tiny lip, so could I try not to push. I did try panting but could not help pushing a bit. Soon after, the SHO confirmed what I already knew. It was time to push. I was told I had an hour to get the baby's head well down. Again, this didn't even bother me. I asked for the lights to be dimmed as much as possible. The bed was raised, and I leaned onto it, eyes closed, TENS and gas & air on the bed.

I found it hard to switch from trying NOT to push to trying to push. Also, everything I read suggested that the most likely time I would rupture would be during second stage. My piles were bad before labour, and I knew they would get worse. So my pushing started tentatively. In my head, I kept hearing "down and out, down and out".

I began to get into it more, began to feel that shuddering power going through me. I was noisy: not screaming, but kind of bellowing! If I lost touch with the gas & air mouthpiece or my TENS I would yell "where is it?" and poor DH would be scrambling around the bed. I also asked him to support my rear end with a flannel. It meant he was right behind me, really close, and it was fantastic. When Julie suggested I stop using the gas & air I thought "What, are you mad? I am totally relying on this!" but when I found the courage to let the mouthpiece go, I made much more progress.

The hour had passed, and the doctors returned. Julie showed them that the baby's head was moving down well. They went away, appeased. I felt my baby's head moving down until it felt like it was sitting in my bottom. I knew we were so nearly there. Julie grabbed gloves, made a nest on the floor, and called the paediatrician.

Finally, I really felt my baby's head there. I remember thinking "so THIS is crowning!" I felt everything stretching but managed to roar and push through it. A couple more pushes, and the head was out. I really could not look down. I was still focusing so hard on what I was doing. Julie asked that I push really hard with the next contraction. I gave it everything, and suddenly, our child was here. DH told me she was a girl, and finally I could look. She was perfect, absolutely filthy, but perfect! DH cut the cord. We had planned to wait until it stopped pulsating, but we knew she needed attention. For the first time, I could WALK over to be with her, I was able to see everything that happened. They took a lot of brown gunk out of our daughter, but she was fine: APGARs of 7 then 9. She was calm, awake, beautiful.

I had agreed to the injection for third stage. I knew that if I achieved a vaginal birth, I wasn't going to care much how the placenta came. For the first time, I had a good look at it. Then Jenna Lily was in my arms. I felt wonderful. Completely elated, and without any of those revolting drugs pumping round my body. Jenna was weighed about an hour later, and despite having passed tons of meconium, she weighed 10lbs 2.5oz. I spent the night gazing at her, totally unable to sleep, in awe of what we had done.

– **Rach Pritchard**

Against Medical Advice, An Underwater Home VBAC

My first daughter, Freya, should have been born at home. Instead, I was abandoned by my community midwife and a most unnecessary, traumatic and unwanted violation of my body took place purely for a breech presentation. I suffered post trauma syndrome and depression for over a year, and flash backs that left me weepy and terrified still occurred during my last pregnancy. In addition, the depression put a great strain on both relationships and friendships.

To this day, I still cannot cope with the attitude "you've got a healthy baby, be grateful...". The strength of these emotions left me feeling frightened and isolated. I sought help by contacting my local NCT group, VBAC and AIMS. Michelle, Linda and Beverley took me seriously and were angry about my treatment. Finally feeling less alienated I read everything I could lay my hands on: *Who's Having Your Baby?*, *Silent Knife*, *Spiritual Midwifery*, etc, etc.

I had started to find out policies on VBAC when I became pregnant. We got the usual responses; basically continuous EFM, drip set up, starvation and to come to hospital as soon as I started labour. There might be room for some negotiation, but not much.

These responses reaffirmed my distrust of hospitals. I booked myself under the care of the Homebirth Team. When I expressed my worries to my named midwife, she said that I must meet all the members of the team and decide who I wanted. Her main concern was to ensure that I had the best possible experience this time round. I grilled each one on their feelings about VBAC. They all knew what I had been through. I chose Alex. All my care took place in my own home.

This pregnancy was very different to the first. I had a lot of pain around the scar area during the first 16 weeks. I swung from cheerful optimism about this homebirth to worries about having to go into hospital and the occasional doubt (for the first time ever) about my body's ability to give birth, something I had yet to do. Close friends maintained quiet certainty that this time I would give birth. Jan promised to be with me and to not let any one treat me like I had been treated before. I needed this kind of labour support.

I took friends' advice and kept my distance from anyone with negative attitudes towards my plans. My baby turned to a posterior position and I told people about my fears, and was surprised and relieved to hear how many had given birth to, babies who were posterior. This helped prepare me for "back ache" labour.

Birth After Caesarean

I reached 37 weeks and the Midwife Supervisor wanted to come and visit me. I knew about her visits to VBAC mums. In line with hospital policy she had to warn us about the dangers of a home birth after a c/section. I wish they would balance the story and warn women about the dangers of hospital births. I refused her request.

Ten days after my due date I ate a remarkably small evening meal and went straight to bed. I woke at 9pm and did something very strange (for me). I sat down in our kitchen and started some hand sewing. Deep inside I knew that my labour had started. I returned to bed to get some sleep. By midnight I had spent half an hour on the loo with diarrhoea and a very niggly back. This was a very different start to my first labour. I sought out Jan, who was staying with us. She rubbed my back and hugged me, suggesting that I try and get some sleep.

I wandered about, and returned to the loo. More diarrhoea and pushing. The toilet seat began to annoy me, so I ran a bath. An hour later I went back to bed. It hurt to lie down. Marco got the bean bag and rubbed my back. I eventually gave up and returned to the loo. I tried to relax and find ways of dealing with the backache. I was not comfortable on the toilet so I squatted on Freya's potty. I could not feel a single contraction. The backache began to feel like my vertebrae were being slowly wrenched apart.

At 4am I asked Marco to get up and get the front room ready and ran another bath. This did not help, I could not get comfortable and there was not enough space to move around in and I felt even more irritated. I got out, squatted as the back pain intensified and realised that I was pushing, I could feel a solid lump. I did a self-internal. The head, and less than 2 inches from the opening of my vagina. I ordered Marco to get the midwife. He asked if I was sure, as we had decided not to call her until the last moment. I was feeling so much pain that if I was only 4 or 5 cms dilated, I wanted support to cope with it and maybe the midwife would know different positions to help me cope. I joked about wanting my epidural now!

Marco could not find the number. In my mind, I knew exactly what to do, but my mouth did not engage. My body had more important matters on which to concentrate and I was already in a world of my own. I walked into our front room to find the pool half filled. At this stage, I just wanted to curl up and go to sleep. This did not work as my back felt sharp stabs, so I slipped into the pool. Bliss!

AIMS — Association for Improvements in the Maternity Services

I heard and felt a "pop" as relief spread through my body. White lumps of vernix bobbed and danced on the water. I felt a very strong urge to push and returned to the loo. Nothing happened, except the backache got worse. The backaches and pushing down were coming in surging waves, and I squatted into each peak. By this stage, I had given up trying to keep quiet, and moaned and screamed when I needed to. This helped! I looked at my belly and saw the four kicks I could feel arrive in a straight line along my Linea Nigra from the top downwards. I felt my baby saying "I'm O.K. Mamma, I'm on my way". Julia arrived and came straight to me. She asked where it hurt and did I want a massage? She touched my back and I snapped "Don't touch me. Hurts!" And she didn't. I felt comfortable with her being in our home.

I finally decided to return to the pool and asked Julia to do an internal. She patiently waited whilst I found a comfortable position. I did not feel a thing. The complete opposite from my hospital experience. With a deep smile and tranquil voice she said "I can't feel the cervix...It's all down to you now". I knew there was a reason for all that pushing. I got back into the pool. The water didn't take the pain away, rather it softened the sharpness. I did not want any eye contact, and none was needed. Marco had asked me to try not to make too much noise in case it frightened Freya. When she did finally wake up, she playfully roared back at me as my attempt to sing ahhhhhhhh rose to an arrrrgggggggghhhhhhh!!

I barked at Marco to join me. I called out for Jan, who came down with her daughter Saskia. The girls played with, and around the pool. I heard them playing but was almost oblivious to what was going on beyond me. Julia occasionally asked to listen to the baby's heart with the pinard. When I could not cope with Marco raising me, she left me alone. No forcing the issue or spouting hospital policy like it was the law of the land.

Sandra, the 'back up' midwife arrived. I remember feeling the head with my hand. There really was no going back. I was feeling impatient, but it hurt so much I cried; "I can't do this, I've had enough. I want to go home". I understood and enjoyed the glorious absurdity of this, with the two midwives gently telling me how well I was doing. Photos show me relaxed and smiling between contractions! I stood up and leaned on the side of the pool. Julia said that if I wanted to give birth standing up it would be better to get out, or I would have to be standing up completely so that they could catch the baby. I immediately slid down into the safety of the water. No one was holding my baby this time before me.

The doorbell rang; it was the postman with a parcel for our new baby. I said that I was hungry,

Julia gave me a dextrose tablet, someone talked about getting a banana, and I drank more water. No enforced starvation. Within half an hour my perineum felt like a ring of fire. I knew the head was "crowning" and I was wanting to really push and at the same time hold back. I knelt upright on one knee, with a vague awareness of Julia saying; "Pant, it will slow the descent of the head". No way could I finally hold back.

I looked down and saw a dark head. My arms instinctively reached down and lifted my daughter from between my thighs up to my breast. She was perfect. A huge swelling on her head from the long second stage did not worry or surprise me in the slightest. No one took my baby from me, no one unexpectedly sedated me. Zsofia's eyes were wide open and serenely looking around. No terrified screams from my baby. Beautiful tranquillity. I had instantly forgotten the "pain". It was not there. Still in the pool I rang my mother. "I've done it mum, I've just given birth to our second daughter". I was not stranded in a strange bed, alone, frightened, unable to move or contact people. I felt so calm, so elated, so whole.

Freya joined us in the pool. Tandem nursing soon began. Jan came in with champagne and Sandra gave me hot buttery toast, smiling as she said, "I remembered your birth plan". No pleading for breakfast! And no pain in my body from the weight of the food.

Cotton cord had been boiled, which Marco used to tie the umbilical cord, before cutting it. Minutes later I pushed the placenta out. I laughed as I chased this amazing organ around the pool! Sandra and Julia then helped me to the bathroom where a bath was run using some wonderful aromatherapy oil. No being made to walk, knickerless and squeezing a sanitary towel between my legs, unsupported, to a cold hospital washroom with toilet bag in hand, attached to a drip, catheter and drain bag. Back in bed, Julia checked me over. I had a slight tear that did not require stitches.

I still could not get over the wonderful care and kindness of my midwives. Sandra asked if I would like the baby weighed. My pelvis, that had been declared as unproven to risk a 7lb 3oz baby, had accommodated 9lbs and 1oz of beautiful baby. My scar was finally mentioned as Julia looked at it and asked how it felt. Fine. I am the first VBAC they had attended at home. I am so, so happy. My second stage began around 5.30am, making my second stage 4 hours in length. Would I have ended up with forceps, or worse still, another c/section had I been in hospital? I believe so.

It takes time to recover from a baby's birth, no matter how they arrive into this world. I was surprised at how tired I was. But this time I enjoyed my recovery. No drugs, nothing to prove and a continuity of care in my own home that made me feel special and cherished. No nightmares, no depression. For the first time since Freya's birth I began to feel normal.

– Caroline L Spear

A Triumph of Hope over Experience –
A Home Water Birth after Three Caesareans

All births are a triumph in some measure. Twelve years ago when I awoke from general anaesthetic to find my daughter at my breast I felt a sense of awed wonder at the creature my body had produced. In the days, weeks, months that followed I started to wonder, to regret, to blame myself for the "failure" I felt myself to be for needing a caesarean. It has been a long and rocky road, a journey of mind, body and spirit to the birth of Fergus.

Two more births came after that first one. In the preparation for Kieran's birth I had attended NCT classes and had laid some feelings to rest, but I still needed to believe that the medical profession knew better, I still believed I was safest in their control. I slid helplessly down the cascade of intervention from induction to epidural to ventouse to emergency section.

We joked, Raymond and I, somewhat flippantly to mask the pain, that whilst we grew beautiful babies we just couldn't birth them. Yet somewhere inside I knew that wasn't true and I embarked on antenatal teacher training hoping that there was an answer to the "why?" questions that plagued me.

By the time I was pregnant with Carys I had some answers and had managed to work through a lot of the feelings of anger and betrayal that those answers had brought. Yet still, as I planned for VBA2C I felt like a bit of a naughty child for daring to decline the consultant's advice to "just" have another caesarean.

I knew the evidence was on my side but that pregnancy seemed to be a long and painful battle with my fear and doubt. I hoped but I didn't quite dare believe that I could do this. Told at 40 weeks that I had all the signs of pre-eclampsia I couldn't hold out any longer and had a calm and resigned caesarean, which in many ways was a lovely experience.

Birth After Caesarean

We decided not to have any more children and I accepted that I would never really know what it felt like to birth a baby.

When I found I was pregnant for the fourth time, there was never any question of how I intended to give birth. My ongoing work as an antenatal teacher, my contacts both within AIMS, the NCT and the midwifery world, everything I knew about VBAC made me certain that birth after three caesareans was not only safe but possible. I also knew deeply and instinctively that I needed to be at home and I needed a wise woman to be with me.

To be fair, I didn't reject the NHS out of hand but I know how the community midwifery system works locally and I knew that whilst my local midwife might support my plans there was no guarantee that she would be available when I gave birth.

My fear was never that I would have a uterine rupture but only that I would have panic stricken birth attendants who would be wanting to transfer me, or inexperienced birth attendants who wouldn't know how to spot an impending problem. Above all else this was about having a healthy baby not scoring points in some birth trial.

I knew of the independent midwife, Mary Cronk from email groups I was on and by reputation. Experienced in the more unusual types of birth at home, breech, twins, VBAC she is practical, down to earth, bolshy about uninformed medics, but knowledgeable about when to use medical care and right on my doorstep.

I resented having to pay for her care, not because I begrudge her one penny piece of it, but because I believe this sort of care should be available to every women as part of our healthcare system. Raymond was horrified by the expense but accepted that only this way could we relax and get on with this pregnancy and birth, secure in the knowledge that our midwife was both experienced, confident and one hundred percent on our side.

So many times we were asked by friends and family "So what does your doctor think about this?" I realised how far I had come in my journey that I was amused rather than defensive about this. "We haven't asked." I would reply.

Although by now convinced that I had not been truly pre-eclamptic in my last pregnancy, I wanted to keep my weight down and avoid any possible complications, so I restrained my lifelong devotion to chocolate and tried very hard to like salads.

AIMS — Association for Improvements in the Maternity Services

I hoped and I waited and I spent a lot of time on email support groups, drawing inspiration and comfort from others all round the country who had homebirthed and VBAC'd or were planning to. I prayed a lot too.

As the pregnancy reached term, and beyond, I was conscious of so many people wishing me well, praying for me. Sometimes in the middle of the night I did wonder if I was totally mad and if I was going to die or to cause my baby's death but these doubts were very rare. I still wasn't sure that the damage done by the sections wouldn't prevent this birth being straightforward but I was sure that I believed I could do it.

There are advantages to being an antenatal teacher when you are planning on giving birth. I already had a birthing ball, Tens machine, homeopathic kit, aromatherapy oils and burner and a wheat filled pillow and various bits of massage paraphernalia. I filled our dining room with candles, I spent hours choosing music and ommed my way through every relaxation tape in my library.

The birthing pool was up and ready at 37 weeks just in case baby should defy all previous experience and be early. We had chosen one with a heater and filter so that it could be left fully filled and I used it to wallow away my pregnancy aches and pains and dream about birthing in it. I ruthlessly refused all pleas from the kids to jump in and splash about – this was my space. Once a week Raymond drained, cleaned and refilled it while I paced about anxiously hoping I wasn't going to go into sudden labour.

Not that I believed I would. Both of my previous labours had been long and slow, I couldn't believe this would be any different especially as my uterus had three scars to contend with which, Mary warned me, might take a while to get going with strong efficient contractions.

So I was somewhat bemused to get up one Monday morning, after a night of mild period type pains, to find I was having quite strong contractions every five minutes. Hang on a minute...what happened to the mild, infrequent every twenty minutes or so that I tell my couples about? "Every labour is different" I told myself, hiding behind the fridge/freezer so the kids wouldn't see me breathing through the contractions. But secretly I was more than a little miffed that I seemed to be in so much pain so fast as I fully expected this to go on for twelve hours plus.

We got the kids ready for school without revealing that I was in early labour. Emma was starting SATS that day and I didn't want her to worry. Carys and Kieran on the other hand, given one hint that baby was on its way would have point blank refused to go to school. Not that they were that bothered by the baby, they just wanted the presents they knew were waiting for them on his arrival!

I slipped away to phone Mary. I was now somewhere between eleven and eighteen days overdue and Mary was due to speak at RCM [Royal College of Midwives] conference that day. She had reluctantly handed over my care to her colleague, Andrya, but I knew she would want to know that it was finally happening. I then phoned Andrya and was mildly disappointed that she planned to be with me about half past ten. I wasn't sure that I could cope another two hours with just Raymond. But I was sure that it would be many hours yet before baby arrived so just got on with breathing my way through the next contraction and willing the children to go to school soon so that I could make some noise. As they left the house I slumped over my birthing ball with a grateful "Ooooh!"

A friend, forewarned by Raymond, came and sat with me while he did the school run. By the time he came back things had kicked on a gear and I was really needing to concentrate hard on my breathing and rocking over the birth ball.

The Tesco order arrived – in retrospect I thanked God it was at the beginning of the delivery slot and not at the end or the poor man would have been greeted with a lot of noise – as it was I wonder if he was bemused by the sound of groaning female emitting from the house!

Raymond rang Mary who was making a last visit to a client before leaving for conference and she offered to come over and be with us until Andrya and second midwife Sue could get here. It was lovely to see Mary after all, I had been feeling so sad that after all our work together during the pregnancy, she would not be at the birth.

It's such a strange experience knowing so much about birth and then actually doing it. I had by now abandoned the birthing ball and was pacing about the living room, stopping only to grab for the mantelpiece and rocking my pelvis through a contraction.

I now had all three midwives in attendance all quietly to hand, organising themselves unobtrusively. Andrya offered me an examination and, desperate to know if I was actually dilating, I accepted. We trekked upstairs and I hung on the bedroom door handles (thanking the NCT poster for that one) while she got her kit ready. At the last moment I sank onto the bed and she was quick, gentle and encouraging "At least 3 to 4 cms dilated" Yeee ha! Ow, contraction coming…off the bed and back onto door handles quick.

"How do women labour on a bed?" I kept asking myself. This pain was just bearable if I was up and moving, the thought of being still, prostrate was agonising. Yet if I had accepted consultant care that is what I would have been advised to do in order for electronic foetal monitoring to be carried out. Andrya's hand held monitor and frequent pulse taking seemed to be doing a splendid job of assuring us all that both baby and I were well. I knew it anyway. Despite the pain, I knew we were both just fine.

Downstairs again I wondered aloud whether to get in the pool, was it too early? Whatever you want to do, my chorus of midwives said. Raymond's mum had arrived and they were sorting out overnight gear for the kids, as I knew I didn't want them there when I was in late labour. I decided I would get in the pool and sank into it with relief, it was like being greeted and hugged by an old friend, a lovely, comforting, safe place to be.

I found a way of kneeling and leaning over the side where I could rock my way through a contraction and slump through the short intervals between. I started to retreat within myself. Not deliberately, although my teacher bit of me noted with interest that I was doing so, I just did it. I needed to have my eyes closed, to just be me with the pain and the rocking and the breathing. I was surrounded by loving voices, Raymond by one ear, Mary still there coaching me through a particularly difficult contraction. Andrya and Sue's voices becoming more familiar. The pain racked up a notch "I can't do this" I said. "You ARE doing it," the voices said. I could feel the presence of God in the room too, just there, just loving me and comforting me.

Mary left soon after that, withdrawing quietly without my realising it. Yet curiously I could still hear her voice afterwards, telling me to go saggy with the pain, encouraging me that soon it would get better as I started to push.

I heard myself begin to moo and bellow and again the detached part of me thought, "Oooh, Gina said in her birth story that you only do a few of those before you give birth." The rest of me thought I might be nearing the end of my tether!

At last the urge to push started, it still felt far too early in the day to be possible, and at last I was doing something other than enduring. I braced myself across the pool, rubbing my

58

face up and down Raymond's forearm for comfort and reassurance, remembering not to grit my teeth and push but to let the air out and go with the surges. I couldn't feel quite what I was pushing where and made a conscious decision to push towards my bowels as I could feel something there. Sadly it was not baby that emerged but I was beyond caring and suddenly, to my elation, I could feel what I was doing, feel the baby moving down.

I didn't need much encouragement to breathe through the stinging – the teacher bit of me noted that yes it felt exactly like I had been describing for the last five years, the rest of me said "Ooooooooh"! Did I want to feel the baby's head? No I didn't. Far too busy concentrating thank you. And then in a flurry he was out and I was sitting back, pulling my leg from under me, taking my baby from Andrya, leaning back onto the pool. We did it, we did it.

So many times I had dreamed of this in my relaxation sessions but oh the triumph of the realisation of those dreams. I had expected to be exulted, elated but it went deeper than that. A deep quiet "Yes." An affirmation of everything I held to be true about the power of the human female body and spirit. The triumph of hope over previous experience.

The whole birth took less than six hours. I birthed the placenta in the pool twenty minutes after my boy. I cuddled him in the pool while he sorted out breathing and Raymond cut the cord – such a different experience for him too being an active participant rather than helpless spectator.

Fergus Lesley was born at 12:50pm, had his first breastfeed half an hour later and weighed in at 8lbs 6oz leaving his mother with an intact perineum and a smug grin. By the time his brother and sisters came bounding back from school Andrya and Sue had tidied up and gone, leaving us to introduce the siblings.
"Lovely," said Carys, "so where's my present?"

After the birth, I noticed two canisters under the sofa. One was oxygen, one was gas and air. "Do you mean" I said, mildly protesting to Andrya "that you had gas and air here and didn't offer me any."

She shrugged, smiling "If you had needed it," she said "you would have let me know."

And she was right, I didn't need it. The oils, the homeopathic kit, the music all were untouched too. Perhaps in a longer labour or in an alien environment I would have needed that kind of support but on the day all I wanted was my husband, my home, my pool, my God and three wonderful women who understood how birth works and how to help me make the final part of my own birth journey.

– **Jenny Lesley**

If You Do Need Another Caesarean

There will always be occasions when a caesarean birth is necessary, advisable or simply preferable under the circumstances.

Although there are cases where the need for a caesarean is indisputable, in many cases decisions about the best way for a baby to be born will be very personal and will be based on the balance of risks and benefits in an individual case. Whilst VBAC is important for many women, it is less so for others, and it is extremely rare for the method of birth to be more important to a mother than the health of her baby.

> "A caesarean mother would never put her baby at risk – she will always make the sacrifice she has made before if there is the slightest indication that it will benefit her baby. The baby always comes first, the birth experience second."
> – **Gina, HBAC, and VBAC campaigner**

Occasionally a clear indication for repeat caesarean may present during pregnancy (such as placenta praevia) or during labour (such as cord prolapse). Sometimes the indication for a caesarean may be less clear (such as a breech presentation) and while some women would consider the balance of risk to be tipped in favour of a caesarean birth, others might still consider a VBAC to be reasonable. Even where clinical indications appear similar, individual circumstances will be unique, and what will be absolutely the right decision for one woman, may be completely wrong for another.

Although an emergency can occasionally arise in labour, just as it can for any woman, more commonly labour just does not proceed as well as was hoped, and a caesarean becomes obvious or preferable. The threshold for carrying out a caesarean is usually lower in a VBAC labour than it is in labours where the woman has not already had a caesarean. Whilst this can prove a problem in some situations, some women can also see it as a comfort. It is very unusual for a woman in labour following a previous caesarean to be refused a repeat section. Some women feel more confident to give labour a try knowing that they can 'opt out' and call for a repeat caesarean if labour becomes difficult or too unpleasant.

Are there advantages to a repeat caesarean?

The realisation that there can be some emotional benefits to having a repeat caesarean can come as a surprise to some. It is unusual for a repeat caesarean to be as difficult and/or traumatic as a first caesarean can sometimes be.

Just knowing what will happen at a caesarean can make a difference. There is often the added knowledge of feeling more prepared for it this time, especially if the last one was a sudden decision.

Women usually have much more control and are more involved in the decision to carry out a repeat caesarean. They generally have a greater understanding of the events leading up to the decision and have often been able to accept the reasons for the caesarean before it takes place.

> "My HBAC water baby turned out to be a caesarean baby; BUT this time it is OK (not good or great but OK) because I went in with my eyes open, I had a wonderful midwife, supportive husband and I tried everything; the pool, different positions, walked 2.5 miles in labour, homeopathy, reflexology. When it came to the caesarean it was less scary because I had been there before and the recovery was easier because I knew what to expect and what would help (and what would not).
>
> "I know that I could not have done more to birth my baby and that this delivery was one of the necessary ones; the first caesarean left me physically and emotionally bruised and battered, the second has left me sore and sad – a vast improvement! And yes, next time I get pregnant the first person we call will be our midwife to arrange another homebirth."
>
> **– Suzanna, after 2nd caesarean**

As a result, although the caesarean may be a disappointment, it not usually traumatic, and in some cases can go a long way towards healing the trauma of a previous caesarean experience.

There can also be some practical benefits to an elective repeat caesarean. Knowing in advance when the baby will be born means plans can be made for older child(ren), support and care arranged for the days and weeks of recovery afterwards. There is no need to worry about going into labour in the night or over a weekend when childcare options might be more limited.

For those with family who live some distance away there is time to plan when they come to visit. There is time for scheduling an internet food delivery, or going shopping, for those who take comfort knowing their cupboards are stocked. There is little waiting and wondering, although of course the possibility exists that labour may begin earlier than the planned caesarean.

> "Knowing the date for my caesarean was a huge help, because I was able to organise one set of grandparents to care for my other two children, and the other set were able to book in at a local hotel so that they would be able to help me after the birth. I also arranged for the neighbours to feed my cats, booked a one-off cleaning service (as I assumed I wouldn't be getting much done for a while), had Sainsbury's deliver the day before, and my husband, who is self-employed, was able to organise his workload so that he could take time off."
>
> **– Helen, after 3rd caesarean.**

Making the most of a caesarean birth

It can make a big difference to a caesarean birth experience to think about what is important to you about birth and how you can keep some of those elements when a caesarean birth takes place. Caesareans are births and like any birth there are often many ways that the event can be enhanced or personalised.

Opposite is a list of options that have been arranged by women when their babies have been born by caesarean. Everybody is different and it would be surprising if anyone felt all of the things appealed to them. This is given as a list of ideas to help you think about and plan for a really good birth experience.

For example:

- ♦ Women have had the screen removed so they can watch the operation, or have used a mirror so they can watch their baby being born, or have asked to sit up a little so they can see their baby being born. At least one woman has even been helped by her surgeon to lift her baby out herself.

- ♦ It can be a good idea to make sure that the paediatric unit, resuscitation unit and weighing scales (where the baby will be checked over), is in view so that, providing your baby is well, he/she need never leave your sight or earshot.

- ♦ If you know or suspect that your baby may need special care, or if the paediatric unit cannot be in theatre, you can ask to have two birth supporters in theatre with you, one to stay with you for the entire operation and one to go with your baby.

- ♦ You can ask the midwife to give you a running commentary, and/or for music to be playing, or for quiet in theatre (particularly at the moment of birth). If you ask for quiet at the moment of birth then your voice can be the first voice your baby hears.

- ♦ You can ask for the lights to be dimmed for a couple of minutes at the moment of birth. Babies are born with their eyes open so if the lights are dimmed and there is silence yours can be the first face that comes into view and yours the first voice your baby hears.

- ♦ You can ask for your baby to be delivered onto your chest, to discover your baby's sex for yourself rather than being told.

- ♦ You can ask to have photographs taken. Some people like photographs of the baby being lifted out of the incision (others don't!). You can also ask for one of the baby in the weighing scales.

- ♦ You can ask for your baby to be wrapped in a blanket and laid across your shoulder so you and your birth partner can 'baby gaze' while you are being sewn up – it's a wonderful distraction!

- ♦ You can delay having your baby washed, bathed or dressed until you are back on the maternity ward. Allowing you to be more involved or to wait until after you have fed him or her for the first time.

- ♦ You can ask to be shown your placenta and have it explained to you by a midwife.

- ♦ If your baby is well there should be no reason why he/she should not be with you in the recovery room so that you can start to breastfeed if you want to.

- ♦ If you have a general anaesthetic you might want to give some thought to who should introduce your baby to you when you come around, and who (among family and friends) should be allowed to see your baby before you do if you are so unwell that meeting your baby is delayed.

For more information on all aspects of caesarean birth see Further Reading, page 78, for details of *Caesarean Birth: Your Questions Answered*.

Caesarean Birth Report – Danny's Birth Story

Having had two previous caesarean sections, I still hoped to have a VBA2C, but luck was not on my side. With gestational diabetes, an umbilical cord that was not working 100% efficiently and a baby with a transverse lie, it was decided that the safest idea was to have my baby delivered by elective caesarean section.

A girlfriend came into the delivery room with me. My squeamish nervous husband chose to pace up and down the corridor outside instead.

It took a little while to set up the drip in my hand but we spent the time chatting to the anaesthetist and the midwife who'd accompanied us. There is nothing pleasant about having a spinal block but it wasn't traumatic either – 5 minutes of discomfort and it was done. My consultant and I had spent quite a long time talking about what I wanted, and when he arrived with a big smile on his face, my nerves settled and I began to feel really excited.

There were several people in the operating room, but the atmosphere was relaxed, calm and friendly. Music was playing softly in the background, although I forget what it actually was. I lay on the operating table, with an oxygen mask on my face, which for me was a source of comfort as I breathed in the cool air.

I had asked for the screen to be removed. I wanted to see my baby being born. My consultant had agreed with me, so there were no big green drapes in the way. I felt the tugging and pulling that accompanies a caesarean and then my baby was lifted from me. My friend helped me to lift my head and watch. First his little head was held up, his lips were pursed, and then his shoulders followed. It was quite awesome to be able to see my baby, his lower half still in my body.

Then he was lifted out of my tummy and placed on my chest. This was exactly what I had wanted. I was able to place my arm over him and hold him. He was covered in white vernix and a little blood, and I was able to touch him, smooth him and feel him. The room was quiet and still. The moment of baby meeting mother was perfect and was respected by everybody in the room. My friend took a few precious photographs.

After a few minutes I was asked if I was ready for them to take him to check him over and I said I was. I felt in control, and I felt that I had given birth, not just had an operation. After they had checked him, they wrapped him in a towel and gave him to my friend to hold, and she held him close to me so that his cheek rested gently on my own.

I was congratulated on the birth of my son by the others in the room and before long I was ready to be wheeled out to the recovery room and for my son to meet his delighted father. My friend carried my baby to him, and then he carried his son to the recovery room.

There were a few complications which involved him needing to be put into an incubator but rather than take him to special care, the hospital staff brought the incubator to us, which was good as it meant that he could nestle in close to my body and then be in the incubator next to my bed when I slept.

– **Joanna Ashburner**

Glossary

Abdominal Palpation
A method where hands are used to feel the baby through the skin of the abdomen

Abruptio Placenta
Where the placenta begins to come away before the baby is born

Adhesions
Areas of internal scar tissue

APGAR Scores
A way of assessing the health of a baby at one minute and five minutes after birth. Scores (0-2) are given for heart rate, breathing, muscle tone, skin colour, and response to stimuli – thus total APGAR scores are out of 10

Benign
Harmless

Cervix
Neck of the uterus which opens into the vaginal passage

CEFM or CFHM
Continuous Electronic Fetal Heart Monitoring or Continuous Fetal Heart Monitor

CPD
Cephalopelvic Disproportion – where the baby's head is thought to be too large for the mother's pelvis

Doula
Birth supporter who can be employed privately

ECV
External Cephalic Version – where a breech baby is turned from the outside to a head down position

Embolism
Blood clots in the circulation

Endometritis
Infection of the lining of the uterus

First Stage of Labour
The process by which the uterus completely opens

Full Term
From 37 completed weeks to less than 42 completed weeks (259 to 293 days) of gestation – measured from the first day of the last menstrual period

Haemorrhage
Heavy bleeding

HBAC
Home Birth After Caesarean

HWBAC
Home Water Birth After Caesarean

Hysterectomy
Surgical removal of the uterus

Iatrogenic
Problem caused by medical treatment

Lesions
Areas of internal scar tissue

Morbidity
Illness, feeling unwell, having unwanted side-effects and/or complications

Mortality
Death

Neonatal Mortality
Death of a baby at birth or within the first four weeks of birth

NICU
Neonatal Intensive Care Unit – special unit for sick babies

OFP, Optimal Fetal Positioning
Helping the baby into the best position for labour and birth

Pinard
An instrument, like an ear trumpet, that midwives use to listen to the baby's heart beat

Placenta
The afterbirth

Placenta Accreta
When the placenta grows into the lining of the uterus

Placenta Praevia
When the placenta lies across or very close to the neck/opening of the uterus

PND
Post Natal Depression

Pre-eclampsia
A medical condition of pregnancy – symptoms include high blood pressure and water retention

PTSD
Post Traumatic Stress Disorder

Rickets
Disease due to poor diet which can affect bone formation

Second Stage
The time between the cervix being fully open and the baby being born – active second stage is when the uterus pushes the baby down in the pelvis and into the vagina

Shoulder Dystocia
When the baby's shoulder(s) become stuck in the birth canal

Third Stage
The time from the baby's birth to the delivery of the placenta

Uterus
Womb

VBA2+Cs
Vaginal birth after two or more caesareans

VBA2Cs
Vaginal birth after two caesareans

VBAC
Vaginal birth after caesarean

References

1 Murphy DJ, Stirrat GM, Heron J, ALSPAC Study Team. The relationship between Caesarean section and subfertility in a population-based sample of 14,541 pregnancies. Human Reproduction, 2002; 17(4): 1914-7.

2 Suffrin-Disler C. Vaginal Birth After Caesarean. ICEA Review (International Childbirth Education Association Inc), 1990; 14(3): 9.

3 Enkin M, Keirse MJNC, Neilson J, Crowther C, Duley L, Hodnett E and Hofmeyr J. A guide to effective care in pregnancy and childbirth, 3rd edition. Oxford University Press 2000.

4 Goer H, Obstetric Myths vs Research Realities, Bergin & Garvey 1995.

5 Clark, Koonings, and Phelan, Placenta praevia/accreta and prior caesarean section, Obstet Gynecol, 1985; 66(1): 89-92 quoted in Goer H. Obstetric Myths vs Research Realities. Bergin & Garvey 1995, p51.

6 Morrison JJ, Rennie JM, Milton PJ. Neonatal respiratory morbidity and mode of delivery at term: influence of timing of elective caesarean section. Br J Obstet Gynaecol, 1995; 102(2): 101-6.

7 Xu B et al, Cesarean section and the risk of allergy in adulthood. J Allergy Clin Immunol. 2001; 107: 732-733.

8 Madar J, Richmond S and Hey E. Surfactant-deficient respiratory distress at "term". Acta Paed, 1999; 88: 1244-8 as reported in the AIMS Journal, 2000; 11(4): 20.

9 Smith W, Hernandez C, Wax JR. Fetal laceration injury of caesarean delivery. Obstet Gynecol, 1997, 90: 344-46.

10 Craigin E. Conservatism in Obstetrics, New York State Journal of Medicine, 1916 104: 1-3.

11 The National Sentinel Caesarean Section Audit Report, RCOG Clinical Effectiveness Support Unit, October 2001, p46.

12 Lydon-Rochelle M, Holt VL, and Easterling TR. Risk of Uterine Rupture During Labor Among Women with a Prior Caesarean Delivery. New England Journal of Medicine. 2001; 345: 3-8.

13 Tully L, Gates S, Brocklehurst P, McKenzie-McHarg K, Ayers S. Surgical techniques used during caesarean section operations: results of a national survey of practice in the UK. European Journal of Obstretrics and Gynecology and Reproductive Biology, 2002: 102: 120-26.

14 Wainer Cohen N & Estner LJ, Silent Knife, Caesarean Prevention & Vaginal Birth After Caesarean, Bergin & Garvey, 1983.

15 Molloy BG, Sheil O, and Duignan NM. Delivery after caesarean section: review of 2176 consecutive case. Britsh Medical Journal, 1987; 294: 1645-7.

16 Sharma S, Thorpe-Beeston JG. Trial of vaginal delivery following three previous caesarean sections. British Journal of Obstretrics and Gynecology, 2002; 109: 350-351.

17 Baum JD, Gussman D, Wirth JC III. Clinical and Patient Estimation of Fetal Weight vs Ultrasound Examination. Journal of Reproductive Medicine, 2002; 47: 194-98.

18 Simkin PT. Maternal Positions and Pelves Revisited. Birth, 2003; 30(2): 130-32. Critique of Michel S, Rake A, Treiber K, Seifert B, Chaoui R, Huch R, Marincek B, Kubik-Huch R. MR obstetric pelvimetry: Effect of birthing position on pelvic bony dimensions. Am J Roentgenol, 2002; 179:1063-67.

19 Roberts LJ. Elective section after two sections – where's the evidence? British Journal of Obstetrics and Gynecology, 1991; 98: 1199-202.

20 Hannah ME, Hannah WJ, Hewson SA, Hodnett ED, Saigal S, Willan AR, for the Term Breech Trial Collaborative Group. Planned caesarean section versus planned vaginal birth for breech presentation at term: a randomised multicentre trial. Lancet, 2000; 356: 1375-83.

21 Cronk M. A Doubly Difficult Birth, Nursing Times, 1992; 88: 54-56.

22 Flamm BL. Birth After Caesarean, The medical facts. Simon & Schuster 1992, pp125-126

23 Bujold E, Mehta SH, Bujold C, Gauthier RJ. Interdelivery interval and uterine rupture. American Journal of Obstetrics and Gynecology, 2002; 18: 1199-202.

24 Shipp TD, Zelop CM, Repke JT, Cohen A, Lieberman PH. Interpregnancy Interval and the Risk of Symptomatic Uterine Rupture. Obstetrics and Gynecology, 2001; 97: 175-77.

25 Esposito MA, Menihan CA, Malee MP. Association of interpregnancy interval with uterine scar failure in labor: A case-control study. American Journal of Obstetrics and Gynecology, 183(5): 1180-83.

26 Francome C, Savage W, Churchill H and Lewison H. Caesarean Birth in Britain. Middlesex University Press 1993, p72.

27 George J. VBAC Experience. NCT New Generation, September 1993, p23.

28 Chamberlain G, Wraight A, Crowley P. Home Births – The report of the 1994 Confidential Enquiry by the National Birthday Trust Fund. Parthenon Publishing, 1997.

29 Lydon-Rochelle M, Holt VL, and Easterling TR. Risk of Uterine Rupture During Labor Among Women with a Prior Caesarean Delivery. New England Journal of Medicine 2001; 345(1): 3-8.

30 Induction of labour Guideline, Evidence-based Clinical Guideline Number 9, RCOG Clinical Effectiveness Support June, June 2001, p49.

31 Lowdon G and Chippington Derrick D. VBAC – On whose terms? AIMS Journal, 2002; 14(1): 5-7.

32 MIDIRS Informed Choice for Professionals, 5: Positions in Labour and Delivery. National Electronic Library for Health 2003.

33 MIDIRS Informed Choice for Professionals, 2: Fetal Heart Rate Monitoring in Labour. National Electronic Library for Health 2003.

34 Mary Cronk, Independent Midwife (email conversation with author)

35 Cluett ER, Pickering RM, Getliffe K, Saunders NJSG. Randomised controlled trial of labouring in water compared with standard augmentation for management of dystocia in first stage of labour. BMJ, 2004; 328: 314-19.

36 Sutton J and Scott P. Understanding and Teaching Optimal Foetal Positioning, second revised edition, 1996. Available from Birth Concepts, 95 Beech Rd, Bedfont, Middlesex, TW14 8AJ.

VBAC Research

A woman with a history of caesarean section can give birth to a healthy baby in the way she wants, without ever having read a single research paper. An in-depth knowledge of the research may not help you to give birth to your baby yourself, but it can help you to negotiate a way around or to remove the many barriers that may prevent you from doing so, or that might make it more difficult.

There are numerous studies relating to all aspects of caesarean section and vaginal birth after caesarean. Those listed here are just a few. Also listed are sources of well-considered, respected papers that criticise the original research and question the interpretation of some of the findings, together with just a few of the pieces which have been written in support of VBAC.

Smith, Gordon CS; Pell, Jill P; Cameron, Alan D; Dobbie, Richard
Risk of Perinatal Death Associated With Labor After Previous Caesarean Delivery in Uncomplicated Term Pregnancies
Journal of the American Medical Association 2002; 287: 2684-690
http://www.uic.edu/com/mcas/jama_2684.pdf

Critiqued by:

Goer, Henci
VBAC safety: A closer look at the 2002 JAMA study
http://www.parentsplace.com/pregnancy/labor/articles/0,10335,239074_264115,00.html

❧ ❧ ❧

Lydon-Rochelle M; Holt VL; Easterling TR; Martin DP
Risk of uterine rupture during labor among women with a prior caesarean delivery
New England Journal of Medicine, 2001; 345: 3-8
Abstract: http://content.nejm.org/cgi/content/abstract/345/1/3

Critiqued by:

MacCorkle, Jill
Fighting VBAC-lash: Critiquing Current Research
Mothering Magazine, January/February 2002
http://www.ican-online.org/resources/white_papers/wp_vbaclash.htm

Goer, Henci
Is vaginal birth after caesarean risky?
http://www.parentsplace.com/pregnancy/labor/artles/0,10335,239074_264115,00.html

Daviss, Betty-Anne
Study's focus on induction v spontaneous labour neglects spontaneous delivery
British Medical Journal, 2001; 323: 1307
http://bmj.bmjjournals.com/cgi/content/full/323/7324/1307

୨୦ ୨୦ ୨୦

Gathercole, Rachel
Home Safe Home: A VBAC – My Way
Mothering Magazine, January/February 2002
http://www.mothering.com/11-0-0/html/11-4-0/vbac-home.shtml

୨୦ ୨୦ ୨୦

Hannah, Mary E; Hannah, Walter J; Hewson, Sheila A; Hodnett, Ellen D; Saigal, Saroj; Willan, Andrew R; for the Term Breech Trial Collaborative Group.
Planned caesarean section versus planned vaginal birth for breech presentation at term: a randomised multicentre trial
Lancet, 2000; 356: 1375-83
Lancet articles can be accessed online at: www.lancet.com

Critiqued by:

Keirse, Mark
Evidence-Based Childbirth Only For Breech Babies?
Birth 2002; 29: 55-59

Banks, Maggie
Breech Birth Beyond the 'Term Breech Trial'
http://www.birthspirit.co.nz/TermTrial.htm

Goer, Henci
Scheduled cesareans: The best option for breech babies?
http://www.parentsplace.com/expert/birthguru/articles/0,10335,243386_194632,00.html

Korte, Diana
Birth After Caesarean: A Primer for Success
Mothering Magazine, July/August 1998
http://www.mothering.com/11-0-0/html/11-4-0/11-4-vbac89.shtml

McMahon, Michael J; Luther, Edwin R; Bowes, Watson A Jr; and Olsham, Andrew F
Comparison of a Trial of Labor with an Elective Second Caesarean Section
New England Journal of Medicine, 1996; 335: 689-95

Critiqued by:

Goer, Henci
The Assault on Normal Birth: The OB Disinformation Campaign
Midwifery Today, 2002; 63: 10-14.
http://www.findamidwifetoday.com/articles/disinformation.asp

Roberts, Lawrence J
Elective section after two sections – where's the evidence?
British Journal of Obstetrics and Gynaecology, 1991; 98: 1199-1202

Korte, Diana
How to manage your VBAC fears
http://www.parentsplace.com/pregnancy/labor/articles/0,10335,239074_110513,00.html

ಣ ಣ ಣ

Peterson, Gayle
VBAC: Should you try or avoid disappointment?
http://www.parentsplace.com/pregnancy/labor/qas/0,10338,239074_115451,00.html

ಣ ಣ ಣ

Simkin, Penny
Maternal Positions and Pelves Revisited
Birth 2003; 30: 130-32
This is a critque of: Michel S, Rake A, Treiber K, Seifert B, Chaoui R, Huch R, Marincek B, Kubik-Huch R.MR obstetric pelvimetry: Effect of birthing position on pelvic bony dimensions. Am J Roentgenol, 2002; 179: 1063-67

ಣ ಣ ಣ

Further Reading

Some of publications may be difficult to obtain, however it is possible to borrow any book from a public library. If your local library does not have a copy of a particular book on the shelf, it is possible (for a small fee) to have the book requested from another library. AIMS produce a wide range of publications, full details of which can be found on our website: www.aims.org.uk. For a free publications list and order form send an SAE to: AIMS Publications Secretary, Manor Barn, Thurloxton, Taunton, TA2 8RH

A GUIDE TO EFFECTIVE CARE IN PREGNANCY AND CHILDBIRTH
Murray Enkin, Marc J.N.C. Keirse, James Neilson, Caroline Crowther, Lelia Duley, Ellen Hodnett and Justus Hofmeyr
Oxford University Press (2000), ISBN 0-19-263173-X
Available online as a pdf from http://www.maternitywise.org/guide/
VBAC pages available on http://www.vbac.com/chapter38.html
A guide to what the two volume tome of gathered research says, contains tables of good practice, poor practice, and practice that needs more research.

AM I ALLOWED? YES, YES, YES!
Beverley A Lawrence Beech
AIMS (2003), ISBN 1-874413-15-0
Available from AIMS' Publications Secretary
A guide to Parents' rights in maternity care.

BIRTH AFTER CAESAREAN: THE MEDICAL FACTS
Bruce Flamm
Simon Schuster (1990), ISBN 0-671-79218-0
An American question and answer style book which is very pro VBAC after one section, and gives lot of evidence for its safety.

BIRTH YOUR WAY
Sheila Kitzinger
DK Publishing (2002), ISBN 0789484404
Kitzinger examines place of birth choices and the impact this can have on your birth experience.

BIRTHING FROM WITHIN
by Pam England, Rob Horowitz
Pantera Press (1998), ISBN 0-9659873-0-2
This holistic approach to childbirth examines this profound rite-of-passage not as a medical event, but as an act of self-discovery. Exercises and activities such as journal writing, meditation, and painting are designed to help mothers reflect on birth and what they bring to it.

BIRTHING YOUR BABY - THE SECOND STAGE
Nadine Pilley Edwards and Beverley A Lawrence Beech
AIMS (2001), ISBN 1 874413 12 6
Available from AIMS' Publications Secretary
This book details the physiology of the 'pushing' stage of labour and considers the advantages, for mother and baby, of a more relaxed approach to the birth of your baby.

BREECH BIRTH
Benna Waites
Free Association Books (2003), ISBN 1-85343-563-5
Addresses the whole experience of breech from causes to turning techniques to the options for birth.

CAESAREAN BIRTH: YOUR QUESTIONS ANSWERED
Debbie Chippington Derrick, Gina Lowdon, Fiona Barlow
NCT Publishing (1996), Updated edition due 2004.
Available from NCT Maternity Sales Ltd, 239 Shawbridge Street, Glasgow, G43 1QN; Tel: 0870 112 1120, Website: www.nctms.co.uk
Includes practical tips, parents' experiences and research evidence.

COLLECTION OF CAESAREAN AND VBAC ARTICLES
Gina Lowdon and Debbie Chippington Derrick
Available from AIMS' Publications Secretary
This collection of articles is a good starting point for women seeking more information on these subjects.

EASY EXERCISES FOR PREGNANCY
Janet Balaskas
John Wiley & Sons (1997), ISBN 0028616618
Specially designed exercises to help your baby into a good position.

INA MAY'S GUIDE TO CHILDBIRTH
Ina May Gaskin
Bantam Books (2003), ISBN 0-553-38115-6
Covers childbirth and midwifery in a very readable format from the perspective of women giving birth.

INDUCTION – DO I REALLY NEED IT?
Sara Wickham
AIMS (2004), ISBN 1 874413 16 9
Available from AIMS' Publications Secretary
Induction of labour has become a common hospital procedure. This book gives information to enable women to ask relevant questions and decide whether or not an induction is necessary for them.

NATURAL CHILDBIRTH AFTER CAESAREAN
K Crawford & J Walters
Blackwell Science (1996), ISBN 0-86542-490-X
American, and as such natural tends to mean vaginal, but good with much guidance on how to prepare yourself for a VBAC.

OBSTETRIC MYTHS VERSUS RESEARCH REALITIES
Henci Goer
Greenwood Press (1995), ISBN 0897894278
The first two chapters focus on caesarean and VBAC with a good explanation of many of the research studies and why they point to VBAC as a safe option.

OPEN SEASON: A SURVIVAL GUIDE FOR NATURAL CHILDBIRTH AND VBAC IN THE 90'S
Nancy Wainer Cohen
Bergin & Garvey (1991), ISBN 0-89789-272-0
A follow on book from Silent Knife, which looks into psychological aspects of birth.

RISKS OF CAESAREAN SECTIONS
AIMS Occasional Paper
Available from AIMS' Publications Secretary
A collection of summaries of research papers relating to the risks of caesarean sections. These summaries may be used as a basis for further research into the subject.

SILENT KNIFE: CAESAREAN SECTION PREVENTION AND VBAC
Nancy Wainer Cohen and Lois J Estner
Published by Bergin & Garvey (1983), ISBN 0-89789-027-2
An American book which may seem rather aggressive as the American system is different to ours - but very well researched.

SIT UP AND TAKE NOTICE! POSITIONING YOURSELF FOR A BETTER BIRTH
Pauline Scott
Great Scott! (2003), ISBN 0-473-09459-2
Available from NCT Maternity Sales Ltd, 239 Shawbridge Street, Glasgow, G43 1QN; Tel: 0870 112 1120, Website: www.nctms.co.uk
An update and extension of 'Understanding and Teaching Optimal Foetal Positioning' by one of the authors.

THE VAGINAL BIRTH AFTER CAESAREAN EXPERIENCE
Lynn Baptisti Richard and contributors
Bergin & Garvey (1987), ISBN 0-89789-120-1
American book which gives caesarean birth reports followed by VBAC birth reports.

TRUST YOUR BODY! TRUST YOUR BABY! CHILDBIRTH WISDOM AND CAESAREAN PREVENTION
Edited by Andrea Frank Henkart
Bergin & Garvey (1995), ISBN 0-89789-294-1
Looks at how the system causes caesareans and how to avoid this.

UNDERSTANDING AND TEACHING OPTIMAL FOETAL POSITIONING
Jean Sutton and Pauline Scott, second revised edition (1996).
Available from Birth Concepts, 95 Beech Rd, Bedfont, Middlesex, TW14 8AJ.
Discusses possible ways of encouraging unborn babies to adopt the best position for a straightforward delivery, particularly avoiding posterior babies

VAGINAL BIRTH AFTER CAESAREAN
Caroline Sufrin-Disler
ICEA Review, 1990; 14(3)
Available from ICEA, PO Box 20048, Minneapolis, Minnesota 55420, USA or in UK from MIDIRS
Excellent review of the research showing how VBAC is the safest option in most cases.

WATER BIRTH
Janet Balaskas and Yehudi Gordon
HarperCollins (1992), ISBN 0722527888
Written for expectant parents and their birth attendants, this book provides practical information on the use of water through pregnancy, birth and during infancy.

WHAT'S RIGHT FOR ME - MAKING DECISIONS FOR PREGNANCY AND BIRTH
Sara Wickham
AIMS (2003), ISBN 1-874413-13-4
Available from AIMS' Publications Secretary
Outlines the principles of making birth choices, rather than focusing on giving alternative options to maternity care.

Online Resources and Information

The Internet is a useful resource for mothers looking for more information on birth in general and on VBAC in particular. The following sites may help you in your own search.

www.aims.org.uk
AIMS (Association for Improvements in the Maternity Services)
AIMS actively supports parents and healthcare professionals who recognise that, for the majority of women, birth is a normal rather than a medical event.

www.birthchoiceuk.com
BirthChoiceUK
Independent website helping women in the UK to choose where to give birth. Provides comparative statistics on interventions and outcomes in different hospitals.

www.caesarean.org.uk
Caesarean Birth/VBAC Information
Produced by AIMS members Debbie Chippington Derrick and Gina Lowdon who are also Caesarean Birth/VBAC Coordinators for the National Childbirth Trust. Offers research-based information and support on all aspects of caesareans and VBAC.

www.doula.org.uk
Doula UK
Information on how to find a doula.

www.homebirth.org.uk and its VBAC pages **www.vbac.org.uk**
both are part of an excellent UK based website with lots of research evidence which has been interpreted by the web author.

www.ican-online.com
ICAN: International Caesarean Awareness Network
A USA based website with a lot of useful information and support for women on VBAC. Has an email support and discussion group.

www.independentmidwives.org.uk
Association of Independent Midwives,
Includes lists by region of independent midwives.

www.midirs.org
Midwives Information and Resource Service
For a fee non -members can access medical studies on a wide range of childbirth topics.

www.nctpregnancyandbabycare.com
The National Childbirth Trust
Antenatal education and postnatal support for UK parents. Some branches have VBAC supporters and run preparation for VBAC antenatal classes.

www.nelh.nhs.uk/cochrane.asp or
www.update-software.com/clibng/eliblogon.htm
Free access to The Cochrane Library – updated maternity care reviews are produced by the Pregnancy and Childbirth Group every two years.

www.plus-sizepregnancy.com
For anyone who has been told they are too big to be pregnant or have a VBAC.

www.radmid.demon.co.uk
Association of Radical Midwives
'Radical' in the sense of returning to the origins of midwifery. For midwives and parents who want to see midwives practising as independent professionals in the NHS.

www.storknet.com
Has a "cubby" or section specifically for VBAC women with well informed articles and an online support forum.

www.tabs.org.nz
Trauma and Birth Stress
An independent website with information on birth trauma and PTSD.

http://groups.yahoo.com/group
Various Yahoo Egroups offer support and information for both caesarean and VBAC.

FURTHER SUPPORT AND INFORMATION

AIMS (ASSOCIATION FOR IMPROVEMENTS IN THE MATERNITY SERVICES)
AIMS Helpline: 0870 7651433
The AIMS helpline is supported by a grant from the Community Fund.

Chair: Beverley Lawrence Beech
5 Ann's Court, Grove Road, Surbiton, Surrey, KT6 4BE
Tel: 0870 765 1453; Fax 0870 765 1454
email: beverley.beech@aims.org.uk

Vice Chair: Nadine Edwards
40 Leamington Terrace, Edinburgh EH10 4JL
Tel: 0870 765 1449
email: nadine.edwards@aims.org.uk

Northern Ireland: Jane Wright
Tel: 0870 765 1442

Republic of Ireland: Maire O'Regan
Tel: 00-353-21-342649

ASSOCIATION OF RADICAL MIDWIVES
62 Greetby Hill, Ormskirk, Lancashire, L39 2DT
Tel: 01243 671673
Email: mary.cronk@selseypc.net

BIRTH CRISIS NETWORK
Tel: 01865 300266
For those who need to talk over a birth which haunts them.

AIMS — Association for Improvements in the Maternity Services

CAESAREAN BIRTH/VBAC INFORMATION
Gina Lowdon
Tel: 01256 704871; email: gina@caesarean.org.uk

Debbie Chippington Derrick
Tel: 01276 510575; email: debbie@caesarean.org.uk

Jenny Lesley
Tel: 01903 219338; email: jenny@caesarean.org.uk

CAESAREAN SUPPORT NETWORK
55 Cooil Drive, Douglas, Isle of Man
Yvonne Williams
Tel: 01624 661269

DOULA UK
PO Box 26678, London, N14 4WB
Email: info@doula.org.uk

INDEPENDENT MIDWIVES ASSOCIATION
1 The Great Quarry, Guildford, Surrey, GU1 3XN
Tel: 01483 821104
Email: information@independentmidwives.org.uk

NATIONAL CHILDBIRTH TRUST (NCT)
Alexandra House, Oldham Terrace, Acton, London, W3 6NH
Enquiry Line: 0870 444 8707 for details of your local VBAC supporters, antenatal teachers or contact numbers for the national VBAC support co-ordinators.

VBAC INFORMATION AND SUPPORT
Caroline Spear
Tel: 01243 868440; email: caroline@vbac.fsnet.co.uk